ESTROGEN

ESTROGEN

Third Edition, Thoroughly Updated

Lila E. Nachtigall, M.D. & Joan Rattner Heilman

HarperResource
An Imprint of HarperCollinsPublishers

HarperCollins books may be purchased for educational, business, or sales promotional use. For information please write: Special Markets Department, HarperCollins Publishers Inc., 10 East 53rd Street, New York, NY 10022.

FIRST HARPERPERENNIAL EDITION PUBLISHED 1995.
UPDATED THIRD EDITION PUBLISHED 2000.

Designed by Caitlin Daniels

Library of Congress Cataloging-in-Publication Data
Nachtigall, Lila.
    Estrogen / Lila E. Nachtigall and Joan Rattner Heilman.—3rd ed.,
      thoroughly updated.
        p. cm.
    Includes index.
    ISBN 0-06-095556-2 (pbk.)
    I. Menopause—Hormone therapy. I. Heilman, Joan Rattner. II. Title.
RG186.N28 2000   99-044799
618.1'75061—dc21

00 01 02 03 ❖/RRD 10 9 8 7 6 5 4 3 2 1

Contents

· ·

1

ESTROGEN: SHOULD YOU OR SHOULDN'T YOU?

••

If you're confused about taking estrogen after menopause, wondering if you really need it or whether it's safe, you are certainly not alone. Hormone replacement confuses many women today and it even confounds many physicians.

Can most of the minor discomforts and major health problems of menopause be blamed on a lack of estrogen? Is hormone replacement therapy the most effective way to protect your bones from the ravages of osteoporosis? Is it the only way to preserve your sex life? Can it keep your arteries younger and healthier? Do women who use it live significantly longer than those who don't? Does it banish unrelenting urinary and vaginal infections? Will it keep your skin younger and firmer? Is it the best method of eliminating hot flashes, insomnia, strange skin sensations, and the other uncomfortable menopausal symptoms?

Even if the answer to all these questions is *yes*—which it is—is it worth it? Is it safe? Won't it cause cancer or other dire diseases? Should you take drugs that aren't absolutely necessary? Can you get along without it? In other words, should you take estrogen or shouldn't you?

In this book, we are going to give you the last word,

the most current scientific information available about hormone replacement therapy (HRT) and what it can and cannot do for you. You'll learn about its benefits, its side effects, and its potential problems. You'll know the trade-offs if you decide against it and all the available alternatives, natural and otherwise, to HRT. You'll find out about new nonhormone medications for building bone and preventing osteoporosis. And about hormones that work as antiestrogens in some parts of the body and just like estrogen in other parts, so you may compare their benefits.

And, most important, you will learn the facts about menopause and what happens to your body when you lose the primary source of your female hormones.

When you know all the facts, you can make your own informed decision about whether it is right for you and whether you want to take it.

TAKING ESTROGEN SAFELY

This book will tell you exactly *how* to take estrogen—if you need it and want it—so you need not worry about your future health. HRT has radically changed in the last few years. It is safe today. In fact, it is *better* than safe. Taking estrogen correctly—combined with progesterone, the second major female hormone—will *not* increase your chances of uterine cancer. Instead it will help protect you *against* it. It will cut your risk of heart disease in half and prevent osteoporosis, the brittle bones disease. All indications are that it delays or prevents the development of Alzheimer's disease and improves age-related memory loss. It can prevent macular degeneration, an eye condition that can cause blindness, and the onset of cataracts. Most important, according to the foremost experts in the field, it will *not* put you at higher risk of developing breast cancer.

WHO IS TELLING YOU THIS?

As a physician, I see thousands of menopausal women, as well as younger women with hormonal problems, every year. As a scientist, I have been involved in the research behind virtually every new development in hormone replacement therapy over the last three decades.

I am a reproductive endocrinologist, a specialist in female hormones. I am also professor of obstetrics and gynecology at New York University Medical Center, one of the most prestigious medical centers in the world, as well as the director of the NYU Medical Center Women's Wellness program. For 25 years, I was director of gynecologic endocrinology at New York's Goldwater Memorial Hospital where I headed the team that made the first long-term prospective study of the effects of HRT on women's health.

All this does not mean that I know everything about estrogen, but it does mean I probably know everything there *is* to know about it at this writing. That knowledge is what I and my coauthor, a respected health writer, are going to share with you.

First, a disclaimer: We are under no obligation to any pharmaceutical company and have no financial interest in any product. Therefore, the information here is as scientifically honest and unbiased as we can possibly make it.

FEAR OF ESTROGEN: IS IT VALID?

Both physicians and women come to me, as a specialist in female hormones, for information about menopause and estrogen. Not a day goes by that I am not asked at least five times for my position on replacement therapy.

I see women every week who are desperate and miserable because of menopausal symptoms and physical changes so uncomfortable that they can't function normally. But their friends and relations warn them to beware of estrogen—"You'll get cancer!"—and even their doctors often don't have the answers to their questions.

When Anne G. first came to me about six months after she stopped having periods, she was having 30 to 40 drenching hot flashes every day and night. She had severe insomnia, never got a good night's sleep. She suffered from alarming palpitations. And because she had menopause early, at 41, and had a small frame, she was a prime candidate for developing osteoporosis. She was also more likely to develop coronary artery disease and to lose her ability to have normal sexual intercourse by 55 or 60 because it would have become too painful.

But she was terrified of estrogen. "Oh no," she protested, "I wouldn't take that. It gives you cancer."

What she didn't know was that if she took estrogen correctly, she was *less* likely to get cancer than before. The incidence of uterine cancer is significantly *lower* among women on HRT, while the incidence of breast cancer is probably not affected one way or the other. What's more, according to a recent study from the American Cancer Society, the risk of fatal colon cancer is also decreased among women who take HRT.

On the average, women on HRT tend to live significantly longer than other women. They have stronger bones. And they have healthier arteries, lower LDL cholesterol levels, higher HDL, and fewer heart attacks or strokes. They may even have an increased ability to dissolve potentially dangerous blood clots.

More Women Can Take Estrogen Now

Even women who couldn't take estrogen in the past because it could aggravate such preexisting medical conditions as gallbladder disease, liver disease, a certain kind of hypertension, and clotting problems, can take it today. That's because the potentially adverse effects on these conditions when estrogen is taken orally can be eliminated by taking estrogen by transdermal patch, which delivers the hormone through the skin into the bloodstream, bypassing the digestive system.

That leaves very few women—those with a history of estrogen-dependent breast cancer—who can't always take the hormone safely.

Stop Worrying

The consensus today among experts, including myself, is that if you need the benefits of estrogen after menopause, you should certainly take it and stop worrying about it. If you have symptoms and bodily changes that prevent you from functioning normally, you should not allow your fears or your friends to talk you out of HRT. If you follow the guidelines we will detail here, it will not harm you and it may dramatically improve your health and the quality of your life.

NOT EVERY WOMAN NEEDS HRT

Although hormone replacement therapy is safe today for virtually everyone, that does not mean that every woman should take it. Many women don't need it. Some won't take it even if they do. Others can manage without it, perhaps assisted by the alternatives described in this book. Some require only short-term help from estrogen, just long enough for their bodies to adjust to the changes in hormone levels that occur at menopause. Others may need years, perhaps even a lifetime, of hormone replacement therapy if they are going to spend the rest of their lives in good working order.

Anne G., whom we mentioned earlier, is an excellent example of a woman who probably should take long-term hormone therapy because of the likelihood of developing the most serious consequences of estrogen deficiency. Her slight build, her early menopause, and her family history give her a strong chance of developing osteoporosis, heart disease, and serious sexual difficulties, all of which can be safely countered by estrogen replacement.

But another patient, Jennifer J., who has sturdy bones and no family history of heart disease, macular degeneraton, or Alzheimer's, needed hormones for only a few years until her hot flashes and insomnia subsided. After that, she got along very well with the occasional use of vaginal estrogen cream (a topical form of HRT) to keep her sexually functional.

Gloria F., on the other hand, decided against taking hormones altogether. Her hot flashes were so mild she hardly noticed them. She had menopause at 59, which meant it was unlikely that she would develop symptomatic osteoporosis or heart disease at an early age. And, as a widow with no sexual partner, she is not concerned about her ability to have intercourse.

THINK ABOUT IT

You should seriously consider HRT if you and your physician have found no other way to cope effectively with the following problems.

Severe Symptoms

About 75 percent of women have menopausal symptoms for at least a year or two, sometimes much longer. These include hot flashes, sleepless nights, strange skin sensations, mood swings, and palpitations. For some women, these symptoms are insignificant. For some, they are manageable. But for others, they are so bothersome that they make their lives miserable.

If you have menopausal symptoms that are severe enough to affect the way you live your life, we suggest you take charge of the situation. It makes no sense to suffer, thinking you have no safe alternative, when help is at hand. You are an excellent candidate for HRT, and today, unless you have had estrogen-dependent breast cancer, there is no reason you can't take it if only for the short term. Try the alternatives first if you like (see Chapter 6), but remember, if they don't do the job, there is nothing yet discovered that compares with estrogen's effectiveness in relieving those symptoms. See Chapter 7 for more information about how it works.

Osteoporosis

Four out of every ten women develop symptomatic osteoporosis. If you are in this group, or have a family history of this condition, HRT is essential. One of the most important effects of a diminished estrogen supply after menopause is the loss of bone mass, which can result in bones that fracture much too easily and is responsible for the plight of all the older women you know who have had broken hips, fractured wrists, and compressed spines.

Until menopause, a plentiful supply of endogenous estrogen helps maintain bone strength. Then, when that supply diminishes and is not replaced, there is a rapid depletion of bone mass, *no matter how much calcium you consume or how much exercise you get*. If you are a prime candidate for osteoporosis, all the calcium and exercise in the world won't prevent fragile bones eventually without the help of estrogen or, in the case of women who can't take it, a less effective alternative treatment.

Osteoporosis is not significantly reversible. Therefore, if you are susceptible, you must prevent the inevitable excessive bone loss *before* it begins. Because HRT is the single most effective way to do this, it's time to forget the old wives' tales and consider taking it, ideally starting immediately after menopause. See Chapter 10 for more facts about your bones and their future. Use the checklist to determine whether you are a likely prospect for developing brittle bones. And check out the new alternative treatments for osteoporosis for women who can't take estrogen or need them in addition to HRT.

Heart Disease

If you have a strong family history of early coronary artery disease or heart attacks, especially on your maternal side, it makes good sense to start taking estrogen replacement soon after menopause and to continue it for many years. It is also a prudent move if you have always had a normal HDL level but, after menopause, it starts dropping noticeably.

Although the facts are not yet all in concerning the connection between estrogen and heart disease we do know that the mortality from heart disease is much lower for women on HRT than for those who don't take hormones. See Chapter 2 for more discussion.

Sexual Difficulties

It is almost certain that you will eventually have to give up enjoyable sexual intercourse after menopause because it will simply become too uncomfortable—perhaps even impossible—if you don't replace your estrogen.

Painful sex is one of the most common and distressing problems women suffer within a few years of losing their major source of estrogen. It is also the most usual problem, after hot flashes, to send them to their gynecologists. They are usually astonished, however, to discover that what they thought was their own unique problem is virtually universal.

The vast majority of women find intercourse distinctly uncomfortable within 5 to 10 years after menopause, even if they use lubricants and continue to have regular sexual activity. Because of the degenerative tissue changes from lack of estrogen, vaginal tissues become thin, dry, irritable, rigid, easily injured, and susceptible to vaginal infections. Lubricants compensate for a while but, if you are typical, you will soon need more help than that. Some women get it from vaginal moisturizers, which can improve the situation considerably, but taking supplemental estrogen is the only way to rejuvenate these delicate tissues, so it warrants consideration even if you decide not to go that route. Chapter 8 discusses this situation further.

Recurrent Urinary Infections

If you have been getting one urinary infection after another since menopause, you can blame your lack of estrogen. Just like those in the vagina, the tissues lining the urethra, the passageway from the bladder to the outside of the body, gradually shrink and dry, making them susceptible to bacteria and other organisms. Many practical measures can help to prevent and banish the infections, but only estrogen will restore the tissues to a more youthful and infection-resistant state. For professional advice and the remedies for this typical menopausal problem, see Chapter 9.

Early Menopause

If menopause—your very last menstrual period—occurs when you are in your 30s or early 40s, you should definitely consider HRT unless there is a *very* good reason for you not to have it. Because you will be living without estrogen for 10 or 15 years longer than the average woman, you will have an unfortunate head start on the long-term consequences of estrogen deficiency: osteoporosis, sexual and urinary problems, and a higher risk of heart attacks and strokes.

Instant Menopause

If you have instantaneous menopause because your ovaries are removed or irrevocably damaged before their time, you will probably have very severe menopausal symptoms. That's why your doctor will almost certainly prescribe HRT at least for the short term (up to five years or so), unless you have had an estrogen-dependent malignancy and sometimes even then.

If you are not taking estrogen and have hot flashes or other symptoms that make you miserable after a sudden menopause, be sure your physician is aware that HRT is available by pill, patch, and cream, making it safe even for that small subgroup of women who were formerly denied its benefits.

THE BEST RECOMMENDATION FOR HRT

Heart disease is by far the leading cause of death among women. In fact, a woman has a 23 percent risk of dying of it but only a 4 percent risk of succumbing to breast cancer. HRT can prevent about half of these deaths from heart attacks or strokes.

Estrogen protects the heart in several ways. Most importantly, it keeps the arteries elastic and able to accommodate the increased blood flow necessary to deliver extra oxygen when it is needed. It stimulates the liver to manufacture more HDL cholesterol (the good kind) and less LDL (the harmful kind). And it helps keep the blood vessels clear of accumulated plaque and clots.

What this means is that women with a family or personal history of coronary heart disease or stroke would be wise to consider HRT. See Chapter 2 for more.

MAJOR BENEFIT: BETTER BRAIN FUNCTION

The most dramatic benefit of estrogen replacement will probably turn out to be its effect on the brain. There is increasing evidence that it is associated with lower risk of developing Alzheimer's disease, and that it improves age-related slowdown of cognitive function; in other words, your memory. See the next chapter for more about estrogen and your brain.

FRINGE BENEFITS

There are some significant and occasionally dramatic fringe benefits of hormone replacement therapy. For example, women who take HRT tend to look younger than their years. The skin, because it too has estrogen receptors, remains smoother, moister, oilier, and more flexible when it has a steady supply of this hormone. Estrogen won't stop the clock or affect the normal aging of the skin, but it can influence the processes that are under its specific control. See Chapter 11 for details.

This doesn't mean that you should take estrogen solely for cosmetic purposes. It is a drug and should be treated with respect and caution, taken only when there is good reason to have it. But your skin may well be a beneficiary.

Other side effects of estrogen replacement are that it helps maintain the firmness and strength of muscle tissue. It keeps your hair stronger and breasts firmer. It increases the speed with which wounds heal and thereby reduces the risk of infection. It has been found to reduce the risk of cataracts and macular degeneration. It improves mood and feelings of well-being. It helps prevent tooth loss by maintaining the bone mass of your jaws. Some studies suggest it can ward off colon cancer and diabetes. And there is even evidence that it reduces the incidence of osteoarthritis.

WHAT'S GOING ON?

Menopause used to be a secret, a subject many women didn't discuss even with their best friends or their doctors. They knew remarkably little about this normal physiological event and often had no idea whether what was happening to them was common or uncommon, normal or abnormal.

But today it has become safe, even socially acceptable, to talk about menopause. Most women now want to know exactly how their bodies function and feel free to talk about menopause everywhere, from lecture halls to business meetings to dinner parties. With this new openness about a formerly private area of life, they are eager to know about this biological process so they may deal with it intelligently.

The purpose of this book is to explain menopause, how it affects your body, and what you can do to help yourself if you want to.

GOING FOR IT

Growing numbers of women today are intensely interested in their bodies and are determined to remain fit and healthy as they grow older. We are living longer than ever before and there is no reason not to do it in the best possible physical condition. Today a newborn white female can expect to live to 79.5 years, and a woman who has reached 50 in good health may live a lot longer than that. Her life expectancy is about 92. What this means is that most of us at menopause have a third to a half of our lives before us.

If we need their help, it is not fair or necessary for any of us to spend that valuable portion of our lives without the benefit of female hormones.

THE WORLD AROUND US

Society has not been kind to postmenopausal women. It has generally found them ludicrous, unappealing, and dispensable. Partly that's because menopause is rather new to us. Earlier in history, women rarely lived past menopause, and when they did, they were considered old ladies whose purpose was to bake cookies, care for the grandchildren, and mind their own business.

Women have also been devalued at this time of their lives because the rules and opinions of our society have mostly been created by men, with female acquiescence. Men have always made the decisions about the desirability, attractiveness, and usefulness of women, placing small value on those who no longer have functioning reproductive systems.

As attitudes have changed, the middle years have become viewed as a second life, a chance for reassessment, stretching, growing. Most women today have many interests and little time to flutter uselessly around their empty nests when their children leave. They don't fall into disrepair, get fat and passive, lose their femininity and sexuality. As a matter of fact, this is a time when many women feel reenergized and renewed by the chance to begin a new phase of life, often with fewer responsibilities, more options, time, experience, money, and vigor.

That means more of us are greeting midlife, if not with total delight, then with acceptance and serenity, as a time of life when many problems have been resolved, identities have been established, vistas have been widened, and more pleasures can be savored.

In fact, these are often the best years of our lives.

NEW INTEREST IN MENOPAUSE

Amazingly little hard research was ever done on the subject of menopause until only a few decades ago. This important phase of every woman's life has been sadly neglected until now for several reasons. For one thing, it is not a life-threatening disease, or even a disease at all. It is simply a normal biological phenomenon. For another, many of the discomforts a woman may experience when

she is going through it disappear eventually, even without help. And the potentially serious long-term effects
have been definitively linked with menopause only
recently.

But mostly, menopause has probably been neglected
because it is a *woman's* problem. Men don't have a
menopause. If men did have a menopause and stopped
producing testosterone, the major hormone responsible
for their maleness, is it possible to imagine they would
not make every effort to replace it? If it was shown to be
safe, are there many intelligent men who savor life who
wouldn't take it?

Besides, most physicians and researchers are men, the
very people who need not be concerned with menopause
and who may indeed feel threatened by it. Menopause
has not been a subject that has warranted concentrated
attention from them. Instead, it has often been perceived
as a rather amusing and trivial problem, something
women made an inordinate fuss about.

But now, with millions of baby boomers entering their
middle years, large numbers of women going into medicine, the demands of women to be treated equally and
seriously, and the more enlightened attitudes of both
male and female physicians, we are already seeing much
more attention paid to all of the problems that are exclusively female.

STILL ANOTHER REASON

Another cause for increased interest in the health and
happiness of women after midlife is the aging of our
population. There are more than 43 million women over
the age of 50 in the United States, with thousands joining
the group every day. Because most of us will live several
more decades, it makes economic, medical, and common
sense to take us seriously.

PREPARING FOR MENOPAUSE

Can you prepare for a healthy menopause? To some extent, you can. You can eat nutritiously, exercise sufficiently, quit smoking, investigate your family's medical history, and get regular medical checkups, especially if anything seems at all out of the ordinary.

Most of all, you can learn everything you can about what's going to happen when your ovaries go out of business. What you learn on these pages can affect the quality of your life for the rest of your years.

2

IS ESTROGEN SAFE?

. . . .

If hormone replacement therapy can preserve your bones, your arteries, and your sex life, turn hot flashes and insomnia into memories, and do other good things, why doesn't every woman take it after menopause? First of all, not every woman requires it. Second, many women prefer using as few drugs as possible and are willing to take their chances that no problems will come their way because of their decision to abstain. Some are not willing to resume menstruation, particularly when they view the cessation of monthly bleeding as one of the benefits of menopause. And others, even those who desperately need its services, are afraid to take estrogen because they are concerned about its side effects and fear it may not be safe.

In this chapter, we present an overview of HRT's safety record, starting with the cancer scares of the 1970s and including the more recent ones in the 1990s, with the details to follow in later chapters where we discuss each subject more thoroughly. We talk about estrogen's effects on uterine cancer, breast cancer, heart disease, clotting problems, gallbladder disease, liver dysfunction, fibroids, arthritis, hypertension—and every other possible link between HRT and your health.

When you have all the facts and a balanced view of

HRT's potential problems and benefits, you can decide from a position of knowledge whether or not you wish to use it.

THE BOTTOM LINE

The bottom line is that HRT, according to virtually every recent and respected study, has been shown to be remarkably safe as well as remarkably effective. Almost every woman can use it safely, although a few must avoid it and others must use it with caution.

Perhaps it will be reassuring to know that a recent survey of 1,500 postmenopausal women doctors found that 47 percent of the entire sample of physicians chose to take estrogen, almost double the 24 percent reported for the general public. Among the younger post-menopausal doctors, those still in their 40s, almost 60 percent took it.

THE ESTROGEN SCARE

Estrogen was hailed in the 1960s as a miracle medication that would slow the aging process and keep women forever young, attractive, and feminine. Many doctors prescribed huge daily doses for anyone who asked for it, often starting years before menopause and recommending it for a lifetime. Then in 1975, researchers linked it with uterine cancer, reporting that women who took the hormone were four to eight times more likely to develop this cancer than women who did not.

When the bad news hit the headlines, the use of estrogen immediately and precipitously declined. If women were taking it, they quit. If they weren't, they certainly weren't going to start now. In any case, their doctors usually refused to prescribe it, even for those who needed it desperately. Estrogen was declared dangerous, no matter how miserable a woman might be without it. Unfortunately, many women suffered intensely because there were no effective therapeutic alternatives.

ESTROGEN MAKES A COMEBACK

But today almost every knowledgeable specialist prescribes estrogen again and a U.S. Food and Drug Administration Advisory Committee has unanimously recommended that all eligible women should seriously consider it at menopause.

Two important things have changed: Estrogen is now prescribed in very low doses. And, for women who have not had a hysterectomy (removal of the uterus), it is taken in combination with another female hormone, progesterone, which effectively eliminates the potential link with uterine cancer.

The result is that, when you take progesterone with your estrogen, you are *less* likely to get uterine cancer than if you use no hormones at all. You are *less* likely to develop osteoporosis. And if you are an average healthy woman, your chances of developing breast cancer are probably not affected one way or the other.

How to Use Estrogen Correctly

Here are the rules for using estrogen correctly (see Chapter 7 for details):

• Estrogen must be taken in low doses—0.9 mg or less per day of conjugated estrogen (Premarin) or the equivalent amount of other estrogens, except under certain unusual circumstances.

• It must be individualized for each woman because everyone's sensitivity to estrogen is different. Some women require less than the standard dose, while others require more to do the same job.

• It should be combined with progesterone for part or all of each month, if you have a uterus.

• It must be monitored by regular and thorough gynecological examinations.

ESTROGEN AND UTERINE CANCER

There was truth in the early reports of increased incidence of cancer of the uterus among women who had been taking estrogen, although the studies themselves were flawed. In the 1960s and early 1970s, estrogen was usually prescribed in very large doses and was not used in combination with progesterone, the other major female hormone. This practice proved to be dangerous.

Here's why. Although estrogen is *not* a carcinogen and does not cause uterine cancer, its use over a long period of time can overstimulate the lining of the uterus and cause an excessive thickening called endometrial hyperplasia. Hyperplasia is not cancer, but left untreated, it can lead to cancer among susceptible women.

Every case of hyperplasia does not progress into cancer even when it is neglected, but it should *never* be ignored. Uterine cancer always goes through a hyperplastic stage on its way to malignancy. Eliminating the hyperplasia eliminates the possibility of cancer resulting from it.

Luckily, hyperplasia almost invariably sounds a clear warning. It bleeds. It bleeds at unscheduled times or, in premenopausal women, it causes very heavy menstrual periods. If you go to your gynecologist whenever you have irregular or unusually heavy bleeding, you will be tested for hyperplasia, then treated if the results are positive. Do not settle for a Pap test, which may not pick up this condition.

If the tests show you have hyperplasia (a possibility even for women who are *not* taking estrogen), the best treatment is a few months of progesterone alone to eliminate the thickened uterine lining. Early endometrial hyperplasia without atypical cells is almost 100 percent reversible and rarely fails to respond dramatically to progesterone.

Hyperplasia occurs in about 17 percent of women who take estrogen unopposed by progesterone and, occasionally, even in those who do take the second hormone, probably because they are unusually responsive to estrogen and therefore require larger-than-average doses of progesterone each month to counteract its effects on the uterine lining. For this reason, monitoring is an essential ingredient for keeping HRT absolutely safe.

HOW IT WORKS

Estrogen, whether it is produced by your own body or taken exogenously, has the job of thickening the uterine lining. Progesterone's role, on the other hand, is to precipitate the shedding of that lining. When sufficient progesterone is taken each month along with a minimal dose of estrogen, it allows no excessive buildup of tissue that could eventually lead to cancer.

What's more, when you take the combination therapy, you will be *less* likely to develop uterine cancer than women who have never taken hormones at all.

ESTROGEN CAN STIMULATE GROWTH

Although estrogen does not initiate cancer, it can accelerate the growth of a cancer that is already present in your uterus. This may not be a disadvantage, however, because it can mean a diagnosis may be made more quickly. Uterine cancer is a rare disease and, unless it is neglected, has a very low mortality rate. The reason so few women die from it is that it is so easily detected and can be picked up very early in its development. If it bleeds sooner because of estrogen supplements, thereby letting you know you must pay a visit to your gynecologist, it is likely to get earlier attention.

Nevertheless, estrogen is never knowingly prescribed for women who have endometrial cancer.

HRT AFTER A HYSTERECTOMY

Until a few years ago, we never prescribed estrogen after a hysterectomy that was performed because of uterine cancer, even if a woman desperately needed it. However, more and more gynecologists today offer it when the cancer has proved to be an early low-grade cell type and completely confined to the uterus, because the benefits outweigh the risks.

HOW WE KNOW HRT IS SAFE

Many major studies have confirmed the safety of estrogen properly used, including my own long-term study published in 1979 ("Estrogen Therapy I: A 10-year Prospective Study," *Obstetrics and Gynecology*: 53, 277–80). The first scientific study of estrogen replacement therapy ever made, it was controlled, prospective, and double-blind, and its purpose was to identify the long-term effects of HRT after 10 years of use by a group of 168 women. Because they were hospitalized for unrelated chronic diseases at Goldwater Memorial Hospital in New York, the women were constantly available for careful monitoring in a controlled environment. They were examined and tested every six months.

Over the 10 years, we compared one group of women taking both estrogen and progesterone with another group taking placebos. Neither doctors nor patients knew which women received which pills and the code was not broken until the end of the study. The results showed that, although we used higher dosages than are used today, there were *no* cases of uterine *or* breast cancer among the women treated with HRT. In the placebo group, however, one endometrial cancer and four breast cancers occurred, closely matching the national average for this age group. Twelve years later in a follow-up of this group of women, we found that those who had been on HRT for 10, 12, or for the entire 22 years had *no* uterine or breast cancer.

Other studies have shown the same results. Most notable perhaps was research reported over a decade ago by R. Don Gambrell, Jr., M.D., of the Medical College of Georgia, which covered 8,000 patient years and demonstrated that women who took HRT had half the incidence of uterine cancer as those who didn't. At King's College School of Medicine in London, John Studd, M.D., Malcolm I. Whitehead, M.D., and others later reported they found, after endometrial biopsies on thousands of women, that hyperplasia and cancer were 100 percent preventable when sufficient progesterone was taken each month to supplement estrogen.

ESTROGEN AND BREAST CANCER

Because estrogen influences breast tissue and stimulates already existing estrogen-dependent cancers to grow, there has always been concern that it could cause new malignancies or reactivate old ones. We believe that it does not.

A Swedish study published in 1990 provoked considerable coverage by the media when its results suggested a slightly increased incidence (a 1.1 risk ratio) of breast cancer in women after 15 years on estrogen. However, the study involved only a small number of women; the increase was seen only among long-term estrogen users; a combination of estrogen and progesterone was not tested; and the estrogen was different from the hormone used in the United States.

A second study, this time made in the United States among short-term users, also showed a tiny increase in risk. But this time it was seen exclusively in current users who also drank more than an ounce of alcohol a day. There was no increase among past estrogen takers, no matter how long they had been on HRT.

Most studies in the United States have found no increase at all in breast cancer risk for women on HRT, while others, including my own 22-year study, came up with a decreased risk, indicating that hormone supplements do not cause breast cancer.

Dr. Gambrell's research, mentioned earlier, studied 5,563 postmenopausal women for seven years. Its results showed that women on estrogen alone had a lower incidence of breast cancer than women who took no hormones. And that women on combination therapy (estrogen and progesterone) had an even lower incidence.

In 1991, Drs. William D. Dupont and David L. Page, of the Vanderbilt University School of Medicine, published the results of their review of all recent scientific literature about breast cancer and HRT, including the Swedish study and the latest U.S. research. Their conclusion was that "The combined results from multiple studies provide strong evidence that menopausal therapy consisting of 0.625 mg per day or less of conjugated estrogens does not increase breast cancer risk."

Another controlled study, recently reported to the American Heart Association, has also shown no evidence of increased risk of breast cancer in women either on regimens of estrogen alone or in combination with progesterone.

And finally, doctors at the Rush-Presbyterian St. Luke's Medical Center in Chicago and five other prestigious medical centers reviewed all previous studies of estrogen's link with breast cancer. They concluded that there is no evidence to substantiate earlier concern that dormant cancer cells might be reactivated by estrogen replacement, and that any possible risks are outweighed by its benefits.

In 1999, a report from the Iowa Women's Health Study, which followed 37,105 postmenopausal women for 10 years, found no link between hormone replacement and the most common forms of breast cancer. It did indicate a very slight increased risk for some rare forms of the disease, more benign types that tend to respond well to treatment and are less likely to spread. For women on estrogen five years or less, there was no difference from those on placebos; for those on hormones more than five years, there was a minimal increase (1.11) in risk. The conclusion of Dr. Susan M. Gapstur, a cancer epidemiologist at Northwestern University Medical School in Chicago who led the study, was that the findings provide more evidence that the benefits of hormone replacement outweigh the risk of breast cancer.

The Odds for Breast Cancer

- Breast cancer is the most common cancer among women, although lung cancer is the prime cause of death.

- It is rare before the age of 30 and becomes more prevalent with age. Two-thirds of the cases occur in women over 50, with most cases occurring in women over 65.

- Most breast cancer is not hereditary. But you have twice the normal chance of developing it in your lifetime if your mother or sister had it before menopause. But if your mother had it after age 60, you have no greater risk than having had your first child after 25. If she had it over 80, your risk is no greater than normal. However, about one in every 200 women has inherited a defective gene that gives her a heightened susceptibility.

• You are at no greater risk if you have fibrocystic or lumpy breasts, except for one unusual variation called atypical hyperplasia.

• The risk is statistically slightly higher if you had an early puberty, had a late menopause, or never had children. It is slightly lower if you had your first child early, had multiple pregnancies, or breastfed your children.

THE BOTTOM LINE

Most experts, myself included, believe that estrogen replacement does not cause breast cancer, even when it is taken for many years, although it may stimulate some estrogen-dependent cancers to grow. Even if it did increase the risk of cancer slightly after many years, however, the consequences of the increased risk is far outweighed by the hormone's benefits. Excessive fear of breast cancer leads many women to refuse estrogen therapy, which would decrease their chances of heart disease or stroke, conditions that are much more likely to kill them.

ESTROGEN-DEPENDENT OR NOT?

Estrogen is usually not given to anyone with an existing estrogen-dependent cancer because, although it was not responsible for initiating the tumor, it can make it grow more rapidly. For the same reason, estrogen is usually withheld—except short term (less than five years) for extremely uncomfortable symptoms—if you have a strong family history of this disease.

However, experts are currently reconsidering the question of withholding HRT from women, especially young women, who have had early breast cancer. Because the cure rate for breast cancer detected at an early stage is so high today, giving many of these young women a normal life expectancy, there is concern that it may not be fair to deprive them of the hormone's important benefits for so many years.

A study published in the *Journal of Clinical Oncology* in 1999 provides some reassurance to women who would like to start ERT at least several disease-free years after treatment for localized breast cancer. Among a group of 319 postmenopausal women who were disease-free for a median of 9.5 years after treatment, 39 women decided to start estrogen replacement and 280 elected not to take it. After forty months, one (3 percent) of the ERT patients developed a new breast cancer. Among the controls who did not take estrogen, 14 (5 percent) developed new or recurrent cancer.

By the way, women who develop breast cancer *before* menopause almost always have the estrogen-dependent variety, which is a disease primarily of the reproductive years. But women who develop it *after* menopause, especially five or more years later, almost always have cancer that is not estrogen-dependent.

THE IMPORTANCE OF BREAST EXAMS

Because growing older puts you at risk for breast cancer simply because you have lived long enough to get it, breast examination becomes more important than ever. Luckily, it gets easier to examine your breasts after menopause because they gradually become less fibrous and dense.

Remember to examine yourself at least once a month, just after your periods if you still have them or at the same time of the month if you don't. See your doctor every year for a professional exam, more often if you are in a high-risk group.

Keep in mind you are looking for a lump or a thickening you haven't noticed before. Every breast has lumps and bumps and it's not always easy to distinguish between them. But usually a bump that is tender, movable, and soft is merely a swollen gland. A very hard small lump, rather like a hard pea, is more likely to be the troublesome variety. But don't try to diagnose yourself—check out every new lump with your doctor. Meantime, don't panic. Four out of five lumps or suspicious findings turn out to be nothing to worry about.

Mammography Is Essential

We believe, despite recent reports that recommend a starting age of 50, that every woman over 40 should routinely have mammography—breast examination by X-ray or MRI (magnetic resonance imaging)—every two years. And, starting at 45, she should have it every year. She should have it more often than that if she is at high risk or has noticed anything unusual. Mammography can pick up very early cancer that cannot be felt and is especially useful for fibrocystic or very large breasts, neither of which causes a higher incidence of breast cancer but can make physical examination for new lumps very difficult.

The newest mammography machines emit very low doses of radiation and are no longer to be feared as carcinogenic themselves. Be sure the machine used for your exam is one of the new ones requiring no more than a total of 0.6 roentgens of radiation for the four X-ray exposures you will need, and that the facility has been FDA-certified.

Mammography for Life

The older a woman becomes, the less likely she is to have mammography. The National Cancer Institute reported in 1988 that 62 percent of American women over 40 had never had a mammogram and that only 6.5 percent had had a mammogram in the last year. Those over the age of 60 were particularly negligent, although they had a higher chance of developing cancer than younger women.

Why? The reasons they gave included not having been advised by their physicians to have the examination; fear of what they might find out; lack of family history of breast cancer; fear of radiation; absence of obvious symptoms; the cost; and belief that only one mammogram is ever needed.

ESTROGEN AND YOUR HEART

There is growing evidence that supplemental estrogen, with or without progesterone, can protect you against heart disease by raising your blood level of protective HDL cholesterol, lowering your levels of harmful LDL cholesterol, and helping to keep artery walls elastic and clear. It also acts as an antioxidant, inhibiting the oxidation of LDL and, thereby, the formation of arterial plaque. This is the major reason why women who take hormone replacement therapy tend to live significantly longer than those who don't.

Before the age of 50—in other words, before menopause—heart attacks among women are uncommon occurrences. Between the ages of 30 to 39, men have 20 times more heart attacks than women; from 40 to 49, they outnumber women seven to one. But then women start catching up, and by the age of 72, their chances of having a heart attack are equal to a man's.

Unfortunately, an early menopause alters the odds and not in your favor. If you have menopause before 40 or have both your ovaries removed before their time, your chances of heart disease and stroke are greatly increased. Within only a few years (if you don't take estrogen replacement), you have the very same risk of coronary artery disease as men.

Obviously, young women have protection that men and older women don't have and it is undoubtedly a plentiful supply of female hormones. Estrogen, one's own or supplemental, is thought to have a more profound effect on cholesterol levels than any cholesterol-lowering drug yet discovered. Women usually start out with better cholesterol ratios than men, but that changes markedly at menopause when their levels of beneficial HDLs (high-density lipoproteins) tend to drop and their levels of harmful LDLs (low-density lipoproteins) tend to rise, making them increasingly more susceptible to coronary artery disease.

Taking estrogen replacement changes that scenario by increasing the level of HDLs and decreasing that of LDLs. In one study, HDL rose 10 percent for women taking estrogen while LDL fell 11 percent, just what the doctor ordered. Another study, reported in 1993 in the American Heart Association's scientific journal, concluded that the cardiovascular protection women get from estrogen lasts "well into the eighth decade of life" and that ultrasound measurements of the carotid arteries showed significantly less atherosclerosis among estrogen users over 65.

Estrogen has also been found to maintain the elasticity of the arteries, increase blood flow by dilating the small arteries, and work directly to clear the accumulation of plaque from arterial walls and to inhibit platelet aggregation. And a new study suggests that it may also help to dissolve troublesome blood clots.

THE EVIDENCE

Many major studies strongly support the thesis that estrogen has a beneficial effect on the heart. The first important one was made by Dr. Trudy L. Bush and colleagues for the National Institutes of Health and was published in 1983. The research followed 2,269 women, ages 40 to 69, for an average of 5.6 years to find out whether those women on estrogen after menopause lived longer than those who didn't.

They did. The death rate for the estrogen users was only a third as high as nonusers, with the most pronounced difference in life span among women whose ovaries had been surgically removed before menopause. These are women whose risk of heart disease soars because they lose their major supply of estrogen very early. The death rate among the estrogen users in this group was almost 10 times lower than that of the nonusers.

More recent research indicating that estrogen replacement reduces deaths from heart disease and strokes comes from a research team led by Brian E. Henderson, M.D., director of the University of Southern California Comprehensive Cancer Center in Los Angeles. This team undertook a prospective study of almost 9,000 post-menopausal women and followed them for seven and a half years. It reported in 1991 that women who had used estrogen at some time after menopause had an overall death rate 20 percent lower than that of women who had never used it. Not only that but the mortality rate decreased the longer the estrogen was taken. Women taking it for at least the last 15 years had death rates 40 percent below nonusers. In addition, the study found no increase in deaths from breast cancer among the estrogen users. As one of the team concluded, "The longer you're on estrogen, the longer you live."

Another large study involving nearly 49,000 women showed that women who take estrogen after menopause cut their risk of heart disease almost in half. And yet another, this time analyzing data from 1,910 women collected over an average of almost 12 years, found that the incidence of stroke was reduced 31 percent and the incidence of death caused by stroke decreased 63 percent.

A major study published in January 1995 included 875 healthy postmenopausal women at seven medical centers around the country; it confirms all of the above. The trial, known as the Postmenopausal Estrogen/Progestin Interventions (PEPI) Trial, determined that all HRT regimens studied, either estrogen alone or combined with progesterone, significantly raised HDL and significantly lowered LDL. The regimens using progesterone were only slightly less protective than estrogen given alone. Moreover, it was found that HRT did not raise blood pressure or the blood's tendency to form dangerous clots.

MORE HEARTENING INFORMATION

Several recent studies have corroborated earlier research that showed estrogen replacement reduces the risk of heart attacks or strokes. For example, researchers from the National Heart, Lung, and Blood Institute's cardiology branch found that estrogen supplements not only bolster the effect of cholesterol-lowering drugs in healthy postmenopausal women, but also is associated with a reduction of inflammatory and clotting factors in the blood that can lead to heart attack or stroke.

And more. A study from physicians at Johns Hopkins University School of Medicine reported in 1998 that estrogen given shortly after a stroke may help reduce brain damage in both men and women. And more research published in 1998, this time from Robert Rosenson, M.D., and colleagues of Rush-Presbyterian-St. Luke's Medical Center, found that HRT helps keep blood less sticky, or viscous, helping women lower their risk of heart disease.

A CONTROVERSIAL STUDY

The results of a study published in *The Journal of the American Medical Association* in 1998 cast doubts on the effectiveness of hormone therapy on women with known heart disease. The researchers studied 2,763 post-menopausal women with established coronary heart disease (CHD) and found that estrogen/progesterone therapy did not reduce their overall rate of subsequent CHD events. In fact, the women on hormones actually had more heart attacks during the first year, although they had fewer later and the effects balanced out over four years.

This was startling news. However, many of these very high-risk women with a history of at least one previous event undoubtedly already had major clotting problems and should have been tested for this complication before being given hormone treatment. In normal women, low-dose estrogen does not increase clotting; in women who already have severe clotting problems, it can increase it. So can the use of diuretics, which concentrate the blood.

THE HEART OF THE MATTER

We do know that for primary prevention of heart disease estrogen therapy works in several ways. It lowers total cholesterol levels and, most importantly, raises HDL levels. It improves circulation to the heart and acts as an antioxidant by keeping the blood vessels clearer and more flexible.

For secondary prevention—*for women who already have coronary disease*—women should be tested for clotting problems before treatment. Because heart attacks initially increased during the first year of therapy but decreased in later years, there is a strong possibility that longer follow-up of these women might show a significant benefit from HRT over time.

PROGESTERONE'S ROLE

It has been known for many years that estrogen protects women against heart attacks but until recently there has been concern that adding progesterone to the regimen might erase these heart-saving effects. But researchers at the University of Michigan recently found in a study involving more than 5,000 women that the cholesterol levels of those taking both estrogen and progesterone were just as good as those taking estrogen alone. And they concluded that the risk of coronary artery disease was reduced by 40 percent for both groups.

A later three-year study of nearly 900 women, reported to the American Heart Association in 1994 by Dr. Trudy Bush, an epidemiologist at Johns Hopkins School of Medicine, and Dr. Elizabeth Barrett-Connor, a hormone expert at the University of California in San Diego, found that a combination of the two hormones was just as safe for the heart. It not only protected women against uterine cancer but heart disease as well. In addition, there was no evidence of an increased risk of breast cancer. And finally, the PEPI Trial, mentioned earlier, supports the evidence that adding progesterone has only a minor effect on estrogen's ability to improve cholesterol levels.

TESTOSTERONE'S ROLE

Many specialists in the field of reproductive endocrinology now prescribe tiny doses (1 to 2 mg) of the male hormone testosterone added to the estrogen taken by postmenopausal women who no longer produce any of this hormone on their own. It helps to banish hot flashes that won't stop despite HRT and has been approved by the FDA for this purpose. It is also used to increase libido and help eliminate the breast tenderness and headaches sometimes experienced by women on HRT. This tiny dose does not usually affect blood lipid levels adversely. See Chapter 8 for more about testosterone.

HRT'S EFFECT ON COMMON AILMENTS

Here's what is known about the way hormone replacement interacts with a number of common medical conditions.

Clotting

Once upon a time, when oral contraceptives contained high doses of hormones, they encouraged blood clots and therefore heart attacks and strokes. Does hormone replacement do the same today?

The answer is no. HRT contains far less estrogen than even the newest generation of very-low-dose oral contraceptives, which themselves have now been declared safe by the FDA for healthy nonsmoking women up to age 50.

A dose of 0.625 mg or less of conjugated estrogen a day—or the equivalent amount of other estrogens—has *no* effect on the anticlotting factors of the blood except for a very few women who already have abnormal blood conditions.

If you have a history of thrombophlebitis or thromboemboli, however, especially if you are very heavy, oral HRT may not be advisable because you are highly susceptible to clotting and should not risk even the smallest chance of an adverse effect. If you need estrogen badly, your doctor may try a low dose, then test your blood to see if the anticlotting factors have remained normal.

In any case, vaginal estrogen cream and the transdermal patch method of HRT seem to eliminate the possibility of clotting problems even if you are high risk. So, if there is a question of complications with oral estrogen, the cream or the patch is the route to take. Remember, however, that the patch provides complete hormonal replacement while the vaginal cream can be counted on to affect only vaginal and urinary tissues.

Varicose Veins

It is safe to take HRT even if you have varicose veins which, in any case, do not result from clotting problems. Varicose veins are surface veins whose valves have failed. All veins have tiny valves that keep the blood moving on its way up to the heart from the lower body and prevent backflow from the force of gravity. When they fail, the blood backs up and pools, stretching the walls of the veins. Taking HRT does not make you more susceptible to them, nor does it make them worse.

Hypertension

In about one out of every 20 women, estrogen replacement taken orally causes the release of two enzymes, renin from the kidneys and angiotensin from the liver, sometimes precipitating a transient and reversible rise in blood pressure. There's no need, however, to return to hot flashes, insomnia, or painful sex. Take your estrogen by transdermal patch, which doesn't have the same effect on the liver and kidneys. Or for local effects only, take it by vaginal cream.

Gallbladder Disease

Oral estrogen can raise your risk of developing symptomatic gallstones because it tends to thicken and concentrate the bile produced by the liver. That's why many women with gallbladder disease have had to suffer menopausal problems in the past without any help from hormones.

But the solution is simple: Take your estrogen by skin patch and you will rule out this potential problem. Because the estrogen does not pass through the digestive system, it does not affect the liver or the bile and therefore does not promote the formation of gallstones. You may also safely use vaginal cream, although this way the benefit is limited to the relief of vaginal and urinary problems and won't help your bones or your heart.

By the way, if your gallbladder has been removed, you can take your estrogen any way you like. You no longer have to worry about developing stones.

Liver Impairment

The liver is responsible for metabolizing the estrogen that passes through it. When it is damaged, it may not do this job properly and so the hormone can actually become toxic. Oral estrogen should never be taken if your liver function is impaired, but estrogen by patch or vaginal cream does not send the hormone directly through the liver and once again solves a major problem.

Diabetes

Some women worry about taking hormones if they are diabetic but the truth is that diabetics usually do better with estrogen than without. Because the estrogen dose is so small today, it rarely affects sugar metabolism, although you may have to go through a short period of adjustment. According to the results of the PEPI Trial, HRT does not adversely affect the way the body

processes sugar. It's best for diabetics to use the transdermal patch, however, because they have a higher-than-
normal risk of developing gallbladder disease.

Postmenopausal women on estrogen replacement, in
fact, are less likely to develop diabetes, according to
research recently presented at a meeting of the American
Diabetes Association. And they are also better able to
keep their blood-sugar levels in check than those not on
HRT. Add to that the findings of a study by researchers at
the University of Wisconsin at Milwaukee who found
that those not on estrogen were nearly five times more
likely to develop diabetes than those who'd taken it continuously for 10 years.

Fibroids

Fibroids, benign muscle tumors that are almost invariably found in the uterine walls of women over 40, may
be as small as a grain of sand or as big as a basketball.
But, no matter how big they get, there is no need to do
anything about them unless the problems they cause
become more than you care to live with. Although they
are seldom painful and are not inherently dangerous,
they can bleed profusely, cause feelings of pressure, and
crowd nearby organs such as the bladder or the rectum,
causing them problems.

Fibroids are not initiated by estrogen but they depend
on it for their growth, thriving best in the years when
you produce a plentiful supply of hormones and shrinking after menopause when you don't. So, if you have
them, is it safe or wise to take estrogen replacement? In
most cases, yes. Only rarely do the small doses used in
HRT today make fibroids grow. But you may be the
exception. If so, and your fibroids were already large,
then you'd be best advised to discontinue the estrogen
and wait a couple of years for the fibroids to shrink
before trying it again.

Cataracts

A study of almost 3,000 women, conducted by a University of Wisconsin opthamologist, found that those who took estrogen for at least five years after menopause reduced their risk of cataracts by 10 percent. Those who took it for 20 years reduced their chances by 35 percent. There is growing evidence, too, that a diet high in the antioxidant nutrients—especially vitamin E, vitamin C, and the carotinoids—may make you less likely to develop cataracts. It also helps tp stay out of the sun and stop smoking

Macular Degeneration

Preliminary data indicates that estrogen reduces the risk of developing age-related macular degeneration (AMD), the leading cause of legal blindness in the United States, which is three times more common in women than men. The risk increases with age and affects about 35 percent of those over the age of 75.

Endometriosis

Endometriosis, a chronic disease that can be extremely painful, occurs when tissues normally found in the lining of the uterus migrate outside of the uterus and grow on other tissue such as the ovaries or the intestines.

Can you take HRT after menopause if you've had endometriosis or will it cause a recurrence of the disease? You probably can because it rarely stimulates the growth of more migrant tissues but you will have to be watched carefully just to be sure. About 5 percent of women taking replacement hormones have a recurrence. Some women do best with a smaller-than-usual dose that will banish menopausal symptoms but won't reactivate the disease.

Arthritis

HRT won't make your osteoarthritis worse and it may well make it better, sometimes dramatically relieving joint pains after only a couple of weeks. In fact, estrogen may help ward off arthritis in the first place. In a recent study, almost 5,000 postmenopausal women were examined for the presence of osteoarthritis of the hip. Women on estrogen were found to have a 30 percent lower risk of developing arthritis and an even lower chance of having a severe case of it.

What's more, estrogen may protect you against developing rheumatoid arthritis, a genetic autoimmune disorder whose most common time of onset is just before menopause. According to a team of epidemiologists in the Netherlands who studied the medical histories of 1,000 older women, half with osteoarthritis and the other half with rheumatoid athritis, the women who had taken HRT earlier in their lives had a markedly lower incidence of the rheumatoid type.

Another study, this time at the University of California in San Francisco, showed that women with rheumatoid arthritis who take HRT have milder symptoms than those who have previously taken it or never used it.

ESTROGEN AND YOUR BRAIN

A daily does of estrogen after menopause may help keep your brain working in top form, alleviating the normal age-related memory lapses and thinking difficulties that tend to increase as the birthdays go by. Estrogen—in both men and women—appears to enhance brain function by reducing damage from free radicals, increase the density of dendrites, and stimulating the production of important neurotransmitters, chemicals that forge connections between brain cells and are key to the health of nerve cells.

Observational studies lend credence to this possibility. Scientists at McGill University, for example, tested verbal memory in dozens of postmenopausal women and found that, given estrogen replacement, their memories improved significantly. And Yale researchers using brain imaging techniques found that 46 postmenopausal women taking estrogen had greater brain activity during verbal and nonverbal memory tests than the same women when they took a placebo. Says Sally Shaywitz, M.D., the lead author of the study, which was published in the *Journal of the American Medical Association* in 1999, even after only a short time on estrogen, "the neural circuitry rewires itself."

Even more exciting: In a 1999 pilot study in which we are participating, there was a dramatic change in the thinking abilities of a small group of women over the age of 80 when they were treated with estrogen. The women, who had never before taken hormones, had all become troubled by normal age-related loss of short-term memory. The blood flow to the brain increased and improvement in their memories became obvious to them and their families within only a month. The study is continuing with higher numbers of participants and careful placebo control.

ESTROGEN AND ALZHEIMER'S DISEASE

There is rapidly growing evidence that women who take estrogen have much less chance of getting Alzheimer's disease and, when they do get it, to have milder symptoms. One study, in fact, suggests that postmenopausal women who have ever taken estrogen are 75 percent less likely to develop the disease.

In a study reported in 1996, researchers at the University of Southern California found that the hormone seems to inhibit mental deterioration by preserving brain cells. Among the 8,879 women studied, those who were treated with estrogen were 40 percent less likely to get Alzheimer's.

This is a very important finding, if it proves over time to be valid, because women comprise 72 percent of the population over the age of 85, and roughly half of the group has Alzheimer's. Not only do women constitute a greater proportion of this older population, but the disease expresses itself earlier in women.

And in another major study, published in *Neurology* in 1999, Mayo Clinic researchers compared 222 women with Alzheimer's to a similar group of 222 healthy post-menopausal women. Their conclusions were that the women who had taken estrogen for at least six months after the menopause were significantly less likely to develop Alzheimer's than those who had never used hormones. And the longer women took estrogen, the lower their risk.

It is now widely believed that estrogen has a protective effect against the development of the disease by reducing production of a neurotoxin that leads to the formation of plaques and the destruction of neurons in the brain.

For women who already have Alzheimer's, a small study indicated that patients who took estrogen had significant, but temporary, improvements in attention and memory, while those on a placebo did not. Estrogen, in fact, has been found to work better than Tacrin, the first drug developed to slow the progress of Alzheimer's. A combination of estrogen and Tacrin works even better than either alone.

So does a newer medication, Aricept (donepezil), according to new information from a large-scale clinical study reported by researchers at the New York Weill Cornell Center of New York Presbyterian Hospital. About 65 percent of those who took Aricept in combination with estrogen in a study of 603 postmenopausal women with Alzheimer's disease showed clear improvement in cognitive test scores. This compared to 54 percent who took the medication alone.

ESTROGEN AND COLON CANCER

Women on estrogen may substantially reduce their risk of fatal colon cancer, suggests a study from the Amercian Cancer Society. If this is true, the reason may be that estrogen reduces the concentration of bile acids in the colon, thereby making tumors less likely to occur.

Additional evidence of its effect on colorectal cancer comes from the University of Southern California School of Medicine, where researchers analyzed data on 7,701 women, 44 to 98 years of age, over a period of 14 years, and reported their findings in November 1999. At the end of the period, they found that the women—all cancer-free at the start of the study—who were recent users of estrogen replacement had a one-third lower risk of colon cancer than women who had never taken the hormone.

AGAIN, THE BOTTOM LINE

So, if you need the benefits of estrogen after menopause, you should certainly take it and stop worrying about it. HRT is absolutely safe when it is used correctly and monitored regularly. Not only will it *not* give you cancer, but it will help protect you *against* it. It will protect your bones and your heart. And, although it can't stop the clock, it can make a remarkable difference in the quality of your life.

Now let's talk about the changes in your body at menopause so you can make an intelligent decision about what you are going to do about them.

3

How Your Body Prepares for Menopause

. . . .

Menopause is a mystery to an astonishing number of women who haven't thought much about it before, but it is a natural and normal life event that happens to every woman on earth who lives long enough to experience it.

To understand menopause, you must recognize the important role estrogen has played throughout your reproductive life, starting with puberty. When your reproductive years are finished and your body starts preparing for menopause, you gradually stop ovulating and your ovaries slow down their production of estrogen and progesterone, the two major female hormones. This time of your life is called *perimenopause,* a potentially trying time because what happens now is unpredictable and, if you're like most women, you're never sure what's normal and what is not.

Here is a short explanation of what goes on in your body from puberty to menopause. In the next chapter, we will discuss menopause itself—the time of your life *after* you've had your very last menstrual period.

YOUR REPRODUCTIVE YEARS

Estrogen is the substance that is responsible for turning a little girl's body into a woman's, making conception and pregnancy possible. A few years before menarche (the first menstrual period), a girl's ovaries begin to secrete estrogen in response to stimulation from the follicle-stimulating hormone (FSH) produced by the pituitary, the master gland. In turn, the FSH release has been turned on by a part of the brain called the hypothalamus, which releases gonadotropin-releasing hormone (GNRH). After one to five years of estrogen production, ovulation begins, stimulating the production of progesterone, the other important female hormone that together with estrogen is responsible for menstruation. It, too, is a chemical compound secreted by the ovaries and to a lesser extent by the adrenal glands.

The Menstrual Cycle

Every month or so until she reaches menopause—perhaps interrupted by pregnancies—the normal woman goes through a typical menstrual cycle. The hypothalamus begins the cycle by producing GNRH. Stimulated by this hormone, the pituitary gland secretes FSH, which then causes the release of estrogen from the ovaries.

Now the egg follicles in the ovaries start to develop. One of them reaches maturity in about two weeks while the others stop growing, and the follicle is ready to ovulate or release the egg. The pituitary releases a second hormone called luteinizing hormone (LH) in response to the ovaries' peak production of estrogen. The LH causes the egg to be released from the follicle. Once ovulation has occurred, the egg drops into the fallopian tube and sets off on its way to the uterus.

Meanwhile, the corpus luteum, the piece of the follicle left behind after the egg has been released, assumes an important endocrine function. Within a few days, it produces progesterone, which peaks in several days. Thus, in the first part of the cycle, there is a steadily increasing secretion of estrogen from the ovaries, and in the second part of the cycle, there is a secretion of both estrogen and progesterone.

Meanwhile, Back at the Endometrium

Meanwhile, here's what is happening in the endometrium, the lining of the uterus. The estrogen causes the endometrium to build up by proliferating the cells into a thickened tissue ready to support a fertilized egg and a developing fetus. When an egg is not fertilized, however, the progesterone causes the thick lining to organize into layers, ready to be shed.

Now menstruation begins. The lining is cleanly and completely sloughed off as a result of progesterone's action and flows out through the opening of the uterus into the vagina, leaving behind a thin healthy endometrium. And the cycle begins again.

This cyclical process starts to change as your body approaches menopause.

PERIMENOPAUSE: GETTING READY FOR MENOPAUSE

Perimenopause, the time when your body is preparing for menopause, can be a particularly difficult time for many women, although it rarely lasts longer than a year or two. You may have completely erratic periods and perhaps some very stressful menopausal symptoms, although for most women the symptoms don't appear until menopause actually happens.

The Physiological Changes

About two to four years before you have your very last menstrual period—your menopause—you will stop ovulating. Or you will produce eggs irregularly or only occasionally. You have depleted almost all of the 400,000-or-so eggs you started out with at puberty, although your ovaries continue to produce estrogen.

But because progesterone production is totally dependent on ovulation, you will stop producing this important hormone. Or you'll stop producing it regularly. That's why your periods may now be so erratic. The estrogen continues to build up the uterine lining as always in anticipation of a pregnancy, but there is no—or only occasional—progesterone to make it shed on its former monthly schedule.

Now, instead of regular periods, you bleed at unexpected times as the endometrium comes off whenever it's ready, rarely cleanly and completely.

Signs of Perimenopause

When you are in perimenopause, you will probably skip some periods. Your periods may be days late, or a week early. They may be short or long, scanty or heavy, perhaps with clotted clumps of endometrial tissue. Maybe they will start and stop and then start again. They may vanish for several months and then return for several more. Often there is no discernible pattern at all to your menstrual cycle and it varies in almost every possible way. This erratic behavior, almost a mirror image of what happened in puberty, can be very unsettling if you're not prepared for it.

Perimenopause is brief if you are fortunate, lasting only a few months. The average duration, however, is about a year and it sometimes goes on for as long as five or six years.

Some women, the lucky ones, go through no erratic periods at all, but simply stop menstruating one day and that is that.

IT'S TIME TO GO TO THE DOCTOR

When you start having unusual periods, you *must* see your doctor. Do not simply assume you are about to have menopause, especially if you are younger than the usual age for it.

The bleeding could be the result of a more serious situation and it requires investigation. Most doctors take a sample of the endometrial lining—an endometrial biopsy—at this time to be sure it is normal. Then if you continue to bleed irregularly, they will test it every six months by biopsy or ultrasound because there is always a small chance that the bleeding is not caused by perimenopause but by hyperplasia, a polyp, large fibroids, or perhaps another hormonal problem such as hypothyroidism. Cancer, of course, is always a remote possibility that must be ruled out.

So don't take chances. Go to the doctor. A gynecologist is the best choice because this person has had special training in women's reproductive health.

COULD IT BE PREGNANCY?

It is perfectly normal to skip a period or two or maybe more because your ovaries are winding down and you are not making much progesterone. But there is a remote chance that the skipped periods mean you're pregnant! If there is any possibility that this could be true, check it out with your doctor. Ovulation is erratic during perimenopause and once in a while you may produce a viable egg that may become fertilized. Therefore, using contraception is always an excellent idea for at least a year after your last period.

Once your FSH level rises to a certain level—40 MIU/ml—which may be measured by a simple blood test, it would be almost impossible for you to get pregnant. But *almost* is an important word, because there is a chance that even though you haven't been ovulating for months, the high FSH may stimulate the ovaries to release one more egg. And that egg may turn into a "change of life" pregnancy.

Whether or not you want to have a baby is a big decision and whatever you conclude requires action now. Go to your doctor and check out your status even if you feel positive you have had menopause.

WHEN DO MENOPAUSAL SYMPTOMS START?

You probably won't have major menopausal symptoms during this preliminary period, the perimenopause. Usually, these begin only after you have stopped menstruating forever. But in 15 to 20 percent of women, the typical menopausal symptoms (see Chapter 5), perhaps accompanied by noticeable mood swings similar to premenstrual tension, begin during this time of irregular periods. Although vaginal dryness becomes more apparent after menopause, it too may start to develop now.

NO HRT NOW

No matter how severe your hot flashes or other symptoms may be during perimenopause, we do do not recommend starting hormone replacement therapy now, except under the close supervision of a gynecologist who carefully monitors the state of your uterine lining. That's because you may be producing tremendous amounts of estrogen at least occasionally as your body tries to stimulate ovulation, and by adding even more, you may elevate the hormone level perilously high. Huge amounts of estrogen can make the uterine lining proliferate quickly. At the same time, you are not ovulating and therefore not producing your own progesterone, the hormone responsible for getting rid of that thickened lining. The progesterone provided by HRT is a low dose, too low to adequately oppose the potentially astronomical levels of estrogen sometimes produced during perimenopause.

Another reason to avoid estrogen replacement now is that slim possibility of pregnancy. Excessive estrogen can be harmful to a fetus.

This may be confusing until you understand what is going on. As the years go by and you run out of the many thousands of eggs you started out with, your ovaries slow down, making less and less estrogen. But the pituitary gland doesn't know that. So when the estrogen drops to a certain level, the pituitary begins to work overtime in a desperate attempt to stimulate the ovaries to turn out more estrogen. It produces huge amounts of FSH and, at the same time, it releases large quantities of luteinizing hormone to encourage ovulation. The alarm is passed along to the hypothalamus in the brain and it too gets busy, putting out more gonadotropin-releasing hormone.

The normal amount of circulating FSH during the reproductive years is below 10 MIU/ml. Now it could rise to well over 40, sometimes as high as 1,000. When the FSH level is elevated, it may fluctuate but it usually stays elevated, perhaps for the rest of your life, although eventually your body adjusts to its presence.

In perimenopause, whatever remaining estrogen-producing cells you still have will respond to the FSH and work at top speed to make more, sometimes much more, of the hormone. In addition, a small amount of additional estrogen will be converted by the fat cells from the androgens, the male hormones produced by every woman's adrenal glands and ovaries.

That's why, paradoxically, your estrogen level may be astronomical at the very time your ovaries are going out of business. Without the progesterone to get rid of the thickened uterine lining, you may develop hyperplasia, an overproliferated endometrium, which could set you up for cancer if it is not treated.

There is, however, one exception to the rule.

THE EXCEPTION TO THE RULE

Although standard doses of HRT are emphatically not recommended during perimenopause, it is safe to take tiny amounts of estrogen now if you badly need them to alleviate severe symptoms. The usual way to do it today is with Climara, a skin patch that can deliver an extremely low dose of estrogen (0.025 mg) a day, providing just enough to do the job in most cases but not enough to cause problems.

HOW PROGESTERONE CAN HELP

If your erratic periods and early menopausal symptoms unnerve you, there are two acceptable ways to get the periods back on a nice predictable schedule until they desert you forever.

Your first option is to take progesterone alone every 4 or 8 weeks, usually prescribed in doses of 5 to 10 mg daily to be taken for 10 to 14 days per cycle. This gives you regular periods until menopause, with each period beginning a few days after you've taken the last pill of the cycle. The progesterone will also ensure that your endometrium is cleanly shed each month and it is often prescribed for just that reason. Many women build up so much endometrial tissue at this time that they require the progesterone to prevent or get rid of an abnormally heavy accumulation.

Progesterone can be used, too, as a way to avoid routine endometrial biopsies. Biopsies are the usual way to investigate irregular bleeding to be sure it is due to perimenopause and not an abnormal condition. However, if the progesterone treatment results in regular periods—with no bleeding at any other time—your doctor will know all is well without the need for a biopsy. For more about evaluating the health of your uterine lining, see Chapter 13.

Some women at this stage of reproductive life are constantly worried about the possibility of pregnancy. The progesterone, with its reassuring monthly periods, eliminates that concern too.

Eventually, when you run out of sufficient estrogen to build up the lining every month, your periods will cease whether or not you continue to take progesterone. When this happens, you will know you've had menopause.

TRY TAKING THE PILL

Your second option before menopause, if you don't care to live with strange periods or early hot flashes, is—believe it or not—"the pill." If you are still menstruating and aren't interested in getting pregnant, low-dose oral contraceptives can bring levels of circulating estrogen closer to what they were before. The newest very-low-dose combination (estrogen and progesterone) oral contraceptives will modulate menstrual flow and regulate periods, getting them back on a reassuring monthly schedule, and, at the same time, do an excellent job of preventing pregnancy and relieving menopausal symptoms.

And that's not all. Oral contraceptives taken long term have been found to enhance bone density and decrease the risk of uterine and ovarian cancer by more than 50 percent. Women taking them also have fewer ovarian cysts and benign breast tumors.

All in all, the very-low-dose birth control pill can be a wonder drug in perimenopause. The problem is that some women can't tolerate its side effects, which often include breast tenderness, weight gain, water retention, and depression, and so must look for other solutions.

So must women who smoke. Today's oral contraceptives have much lower doses of hormones than those of the past, but when combined with smoking they may still significantly raise the risk of clotting problems and heart disease. Research reported in 1999 by Mary C. Davis, Ph.D., of Arizona State University measured the effects of smoking and oral contraceptives in response to acute stress. One of the principal findings was that oral contraceptive users had significantly greater cardiovascular reactivity to stress—but *only* if they were also smokers.

If you do not smoke, don't worry. The very-low-dose oral contraceptives, which contain only about a quarter of the estrogen and less than half the progesterone of their predecessors, have been declared safe by the FDA for healthy nonsmoking women up to the age of 50 or menopause, whichever comes first.

THE PILL VS. HRT NOW

Oral contraceptives *suppress* and *replace* your own production of estrogen, unlike HRT, which *adds* estrogen to your own supply that may sometimes rise to phenomenal levels in perimenopause as the ovaries respond to the pressure from the pituitary gland to get going again. At the same time, they ensure an adequate supply of progesterone.

You won't know if you've had menopause while you are on oral contraceptives, unless you stop taking them for a week or two and have your FSH level measured. If that level is beyond 40 MIU/ml, you are menopausal and, if you like, you can switch directly to HRT. You could stay on the pills, using them as replacement, but they may supply more hormones than you need and HRT is a better choice.

TRY VITAMINS

If your only problem during perimenopause is early hot flashes, daily doses of vitamin E may be all you need to keep them under control. This antioxidant vitamin often does an adequate job on mild menopausal symptoms. Although no one knows exactly how it works—especially since vitamin E is a coenzyme that is not normally manufactured in the human body—it seems to help maintain the estrogen level on a more even keel. Try taking 400 units twice a day and, if necessary, double the dose for a daily total of 1,600 units.

Some women also find supplements of vitamins B and C to be helpful for symptoms, although there have been no scientific studies to determine their effectiveness. If you want to try them, start off with a 500 mg of vitamin C a day and one B-50 tablet (at least 50 mcg or mg of all the essential B vitamins).

See Chapter 6 for more suggestions other than estrogen for dealing with uncomfortable menopausal symptoms.

COPING WITH MOOD SWINGS

For constant and disconcerting PMS-like mood swings during this transitional time, talk to your doctor about the possibility of using tranquilizers or mood elevators until the tremendous peaks and valleys of estrogen production have leveled off. Or try taking oral contraceptives, as discussed above. They may greatly relieve those mood swings.

Meantime, remember that perimenopause is a transient phase that rarely lasts longer than a year.

MENOPAUSE AT LAST

Eventually you will have no menstrual periods, erratic or otherwise. When you have had none for 12 consecutive months, you can safely conclude you have reached menopause.

To be sure this is truly the case, especially before prescribing hormone replacement therapy, your doctor will confirm your new status by sending a blood sample to a laboratory to be analyzed for circulating FSH. The closer to menopause you are, the higher the FSH level. At 20 or 25 MIU/ml, you are on your way. At 40 MIU/ml or more, you are certifiably menopausal.

4

MENOPAUSE: WHAT'S GOING ON?

Menopause is your very last menstrual period. It is just one moment in time, a single event in a long physiological process called the climacteric syndrome. This syndrome is a sequence of happenings that may go on for more than 35 years, starting in your late 20s or early 30s when your estrogen production begins to taper off, and ending long after menopause.

The climacteric includes all those years of diminishing estrogen production, both before and after your last period. At one point in the climacteric, when the hormone produced by the ovaries is no longer sufficient to stimulate ovulation and menstrual periods, you have menopause. Meanwhile, the climacteric continues, with the hormone level inexorably diminishing and more changes happening in your body because of it.

The whole process is like puberty in reverse. All the parts and reproductive abilities of your body that once developed in puberty and then were maintained by estrogen now begin to change again as the ovaries gradually give up their dominant role.

WHEN WILL IT HAPPEN?

The average age for menopause, your last period, is 52, with a normal range of 45 to 55. Some women, of course, have theirs much earlier or much later. About 5 out of every 100 women continue to menstruate after age 53, some even as late as 60 or more. Approximately 8 out of 100 have menopause before the age of 40.

Your age at menopause is mainly determined by your genes. So, without outside interference, you will have your last period at about the same age as your mother, maternal grandmother, aunts, and sisters had theirs.

Nobody knows why the ovaries stop producing estrogen at a certain time, but it probably happens when your ovarian follicles are finally depleted. At birth, a female child possesses approximately 400,000 follicles. By the age of 40, the typical woman has only 5,000 to 10,000 left, and the numbers decline unrelentingly thereafter.

Contrary to what most people think, the age you were when you had your first period has no relationship to the age you'll be at menopause. In fact, there is no correlation at all between these two most important events in your biological history. So whether you began having periods at 11 or 17 has no bearing on what's going to be.

Of course, you will have menopause *instantly*, from one day to the next, at whatever age you are, if your ovaries are severely damaged or surgically removed before they have stopped making hormones on their own.

The Reasons for Early Menopause

If you are among the 8 percent of women who have spontaneous (that is, nonsurgical) menopause before the age of 40, it's probably because you come from a family that tends to run out of eggs very early. But there are a few other possible, although rare, reasons. Some women have an abnormal number of chromosomes that leads to decreased egg production and they quit making estrogen at a very early age, perhaps even in their 20s. And occasionally a woman suffers from an autoimmune disease, causing her to produce antibodies to her own ovarian tissue.

Women who have had hysterectomies many years before their menopause (but still have their ovaries) tend to have it earlier than their genes would have dictated. So do women who have had tubal ligations. That's because some blood circulation may have been compromised in the pelvic area as a result of the surgery.

Heavy smoking can also cause you to have menopause before your time. Women who smoke tend to have menopause 5 to 10 years earlier than their nonsmoking relatives. If you are a smoker, the fact that an addiction to cigarettes can so seriously affect a normal biological process should give you yet another reason to reconsider the habit.

In addition, increasingly common reasons for premature menopause today are chemotherapy and radiation because more and more women now survive cancer. Both treatments can destroy ovarian function and precipitate menopause.

The Effects of Early Menopause

Many women are delighted to have an early menopause because it means no more menstrual periods and no more pregnancies. But premature menopause or menopause at the early end of the normal spectrum does have its drawbacks.

The primary risk is that you will develop the consequences of estrogen deficiency much sooner than you would have if it had happened later. Your extra years without the hormone give you that much more time to develop some major health problems associated with estrogen deficiency. These include osteoporosis, vaginal and urinary changes, coronary artery disease, macular degeneration, and Alzheimer's disease.

On the other hand, you have less chance of getting ovarian cancer because you have spent fewer years of your life ovulating. This is the same reason why women who have taken oral contraceptives for many years also have a lower incidence of ovarian cancer.

Late Menopause: What's Good About It?

If you are among the 5 percent of women who continue to produce enough estrogen for ovulation and menstruation after the age of 53, you have several advantages over those who stop much earlier. That's because the longer you have estrogen circulating throughout the tissues of the body, the longer you are protected against some of the changes that happen when you lose it.

Your estrogen, for example, protects you against heart disease. It prevents you from developing osteoporosis, giving you stronger bones as "money in the bank" for the future when they won't retain as much calcium as they do now. It helps maintain your youthful appearance. It keeps your vaginal and urinary tissues in good operating condition.

Since it takes about 10 years from the time you lose your major source of estrogen until these tissues are seriously affected, you are way ahead if you have a late menopause.

The only real disadvantages are a very slight increase in the incidence of breast cancer and a slightly higher-than-normal risk of ovarian cancer because the more ovulations you have in your lifetime the more likely you are to develop these kinds of cancer. If you are in your 50s and not yet menopausal, it is especially important that you go to your doctor at least once a year for a thorough physical examination of your ovaries, perhaps supplemented by an ultrasound picture, to make sure all is well. Ovarian cancer has no symptoms in its early stages.

HOW YOUR BODY CHANGES

Many of the typical changes that start taking place in your body happen to *every* woman at menopause. Every woman stops menstruating and becomes infertile. Every woman's reproductive organs, no longer needed for conception and pregnancy, shrink and change. Every woman's skin, muscles, heart, vagina, urinary tract, and bones show the effects of the depletion of the female hormones she has been producing since puberty.

The ovaries, once the size of walnuts, shrink to about a third of their former size. The flow of mucus from the cervix and vagina gradually wanes. The endometrium thins and shrinks until it finally becomes nonfunctioning. The uterus slowly diminishes from its original size (about as big as your fist and approximately 2 inches thick) to a third of its former dimensions.

The vagina and vulva shrink and the vaginal walls become thinner, drier, more fragile, less resilient, less elastic, and less lubricated. The membrane that lines the vagina becomes thinner because the cornified cells, which formed a tough protective layer when estrogen was plentiful, disappear.

The distance between the vagina and the urethra grows shorter and, like the vaginal lining, the urethra's tissues become thinner and more fragile. Meanwhile, the bladder loses its elasticity and can't hold as much urine as it once did. The muscles that form the pelvic floor and support your internal organs become more lax, so these organs tend to drop lower in your abdomen.

The breasts lose their former thick layer of subcutaneous fat and their glandular tissue shrinks because it no longer must be ready to nourish a baby.

Every woman loses much of the fat layer just under the skin and suffers a noticeable loss of skin oil and moisture. Muscles tend to lose tone and bone mass diminishes at an accelerated rate. The cardiovascular system loses the beneficial effect of estrogen on HDL cholesterol and the arteries become narrower and less elastic.

These changes that happen to every woman after menopause occur because all of these tissues have receptors for estrogen, meaning that the hormone stimulates them in some way. Without the influence of estrogen, they respond by making changes, all of them of an atrophic nature. The changes usually start to become evident within about three years after menopause, although sometimes you will notice them even before that.

The Timing Differs

Every woman's timetable is different. If your ovaries, along with your adrenal glands and fat tissue, continue to produce some estrogen after menopause—although not enough, of course, to sustain ovulation and menstrual periods—these universal changes will occur at a more leisurely pace. At the other extreme, if your ovaries are removed or suppressed abruptly, almost completely cutting off your estrogen supply, the changes will occur much more quickly.

The End of Your Reproductive Years

When you consider that most of the parts of the female body that alter after menopause are those associated with reproduction, you can understand what is going on. Because your body no longer has to be prepared to respond instantly to the growth and nourishment of a fetus, it returns to a reproductively quiescent state. That is a great relief for many of us and most women today greet the absence of menstrual periods and fertility with equanimity if not joy.

Today, however, it is possible for women beyond menopause, especially those whose ovaries have stopped turning out eggs at an early age, to have babies through egg donation and in vitro fertilization when a donor egg is fertilized with the partner's sperm and implanted into the uterus. Not only that, but your own fertilized eggs—embryos—can now be retrieved and frozen before menopause and saved for a later time. These new procedures can result in successful pregnancies for women who thought their childbearing days were over.

THE TRANSIENT SYMPTOMS

There are other common occurrences in a woman's body at menopause, although not everyone experiences them in the same way. These are the transient responses to the new low levels of female hormones, the "symptoms" of the hormonal upheaval that is taking place rather than atrophic physical changes in body tissues.

The most common symptom, of course, is the notorious hot flash, the sudden envelopment of the upper body by a wave of heat and perspiration. But there are many other typical symptoms: palpitations, insomnia, numbness, pins and needles, crawly skin sensations, strange pains, shortness of breath, dizziness, fatigue, headaches, irritability, and depression.

That's a lengthy list, but nobody ever has all of them and probably nobody ever has most of them either. Some women never have any. But when you have them, they are not figments of your imagination but real physiological phenomena. They are not harmful, but they can make you very uncomfortable and, in some cases, absolutely miserable. Eventually, however, they will pass.

About one in every 10 women has no very noticeable outward signs of menopause and wouldn't know anything was happening if she didn't stop having menstrual periods. The reason is that her production of female hormones diminishes so gradually and gently that her body has time to adjust without stress. In addition, she probably continues to produce some estrogen, although not nearly enough for periods and fertility.

The rest of us, the great majority, will have some of the symptoms. Most women experience, at the very least, some hot flashes and excessive perspiration, which may not bother them at all but are simply interesting to observe. But for other women, the flashes, sweats, and some of the other symptoms may be frequent or severe enough to affect the quality of their lives.

What are you going to do about them? Can you live with them or do you need help? You will find your alternatives in Chapters 6 and 7.

5

HOT FLASHES AND OTHER STRANGE SYMPTOMS

••

Nobody can predict how you are going to weather menopause because everybody is different. Some women hardly notice the entire phenomenon. They simply stop having menstrual periods and that's that. Others find this one of the most trying times of their lives, with symptoms that make it impossible for them to function normally. Between the two extremes are the majority of us who have symptoms ranging from insignificant to incapacitating.

Whatever happens in your case, remember that you are *normal* and that these physiological events are not imaginary. This is a measurable physical happening, with a wide range of normal symptoms.

WHY THE DIFFERENCES?

Whether or not you develop symptoms at menopause is not under your control. It is mainly a matter of the inherited rate at which you stop producing estrogen and the number of estrogen receptors you possess.

If you lose estrogen very rapidly, you will be much more likely to be seriously affected by your changing hormonal levels. That's why women who lose theirs

abruptly because of surgery or suppression by chemotherapy, radiation, or illness, usually have the worst
problems of all. But if you have lucky genes and lose
your ability to make copious estrogen very slowly—
especially if you continue, as many women do, to produce significant estrogen in your adrenals, fat tissue,
and even your ovaries—your symptoms will be negligi-
ble.

Current thought is that another reason for differences
in the way hot flashes are experienced is the number of
estrogen receptors in your hypothalamus, which controls
temperature regulation. Some women have 100,000
receptors eager to be supplied with estrogen, while other
perfectly normal women have only 2,000 or so. When
estrogen production shuts down, the women with the
most receptors tend to have the worst symptoms.

There's nothing superior or inferior about the women
who have mild symptoms or severe symptoms in
response to diminished estrogen. Hot flashes, palpitations, metallic tastes, and insomnia don't happen only to
unfulfilled discontents, hypochondriacs, and women
who have failed to lead healthy, sane, active lives. As a
colleague says, "Women who complain about hot flashes
are not women who are neurotic. They are women having bad hot flashes. And women who do not complain of
hot flashes are not wonderful stoic women of good pioneer stock. They are women who are *not* having bad hot
flashes."

So stop blaming yourself, as so many women do, if
you are overwhelmed by symptoms, and spend your
energy instead on helping yourself cope with them.

By the way, women who have an early menopause are
more likely to have hot flashes. And so, a recent study
has found, are thin smokers, perhaps because smoking
tends to have an antiestrogenic effect and thin women
get minimal estrogen production from their fat tissue.

DON'T PUT UP WITH MISERY

The typical menopausal symptoms such as hot flashes and strange tastes are not dangerous or harmful, no matter how bad they feel. And, except in rare cases, they disappear after a while even if you don't do anything about them.

When they make your life miserable, however, you don't have to simply endure them, although an amazing number of women put up with them for months or even years before seeking help. All of the symptoms can be eliminated in very short order by hormone replacement therapy (HRT), safe for virtually every woman today. If you can't take estrogen or don't want to, there are alternative remedies that may help. However you decide to do it, remember that it's not necessary to suffer because help is at hand. It always makes excellent sense to fight back.

THE NOTORIOUS HOT FLASH

Of all the variable transient symptoms, the most common is the hot flash (or, if you are British, hot flush). Flashes can be mild or severe, slightly discomforting or definitely distressing. Sometimes they are even frightening, although they are quite harmless.

Nine out of every 10 women at menopause have hot flashes or some other equally strange *vasomotor disturbances* related to the regulation of body temperature. For half of these women, the symptoms are gone within a year. For 30 percent of them, they last up to two and a half years. For the remaining 20 percent, the flashes and/or other symptoms continue for longer than that, maybe 5 or 10 years, sometimes even 20 years. Some unfortunate women—an estimated 2 to 3 percent—have them until the day they die. Because the 1970s and 1980s were a time when many women gave up estrogen replacement or were afraid to start it because of the reports of a link with cancer, doctors today see an astonishing number of women who had menopause many years ago, never took estrogen, and are still suffering with flashes.

Many women have only three or four episodes a day and hardly notice them, while others have 30, 40, or even 50 severe hot flashes a day, one right after the other. The flashes are usually at their worst at night.

Hot Flash Facts

• A hot flash is a feeling of intense heat that envelops the body, usually only from the waist up and especially the face and neck. The blood vessels on the skin's surface dilate, often causing red splotches or a rosy flush. In most cases, the flash is accompanied by profuse perspiration, so much for some women that they have to change their clothes or their bed linens, while others merely have to wipe their brows.

• A hot flash is often sensed a few seconds before it occurs. You may have a warning sensation or *aura* that signals an impending heat wave.

• The flash is often followed by chills and sometimes intense shivering, along with a feeling of constriction of the skin that may last for a few hours.

• Several studies have shown that skin temperature is measurably elevated during a flash and that there is a 10 to 15 percent increase in pulse rate. These effects begin just before the flash occurs.

• Flashes usually last for 3 to 6 minutes, though they occasionally endure for up to an hour.

- Some women have a variation on hot flashes: "cold sweats," which are just what they sound like—chills with profuse perspiration and uncontrollable shivering.

What Causes Them?

When its estrogen receptors are no longer satisfied by a plentiful supply of estrogen, the hypothalamus produces an epinephrine-like neurotransmitter that affects the body's heat-regulating systems and causes the symptoms.

The level of estrogen deficiency at which you are likely to start having flashes can vary widely. Some women have no flashes until their estrogen level is very low and their FSH is extremely high, while others have them at any time during the changing biological process.

What Triggers Them?

If you are extremely susceptible, almost anything can trigger them, especially if it normally raises body temperature and/or dilates the capillaries. For example, a flash may be set off by exercise, external temperature, overwork, excessive clothing, fear, joy, excitement, anxiety, or stress. Alcohol and caffeine, both of which cause capillaries to dilate, will do it too. So will hot drinks and spicy foods.

Although flashes tend to occur less frequently when you are relaxed and rested, they are at their worst at night. We don't know why but it is probably because the hypothalamus responds most vigorously when all other functions are in a resting state.

Cooling Off

If you're going to get flashes, you'll get them no matter what—if you don't take estrogen. But if you take some practical measures, you may ward off a few now and then. For example, because fatigue makes you more susceptible, try to get adequate rest. Dress in layers so you can remove clothing when you begin to feel warm.

Avoid hot drinks. As much as possible, try to keep your cool in trying circumstances. Give up the drinks and foods that trigger the heat waves. Be sure to eat balanced meals and get adequate exercise. Check out the suggestions, ranging from HRT to deep breathing, in the next chapter.

OTHER TYPICAL MENOPAUSAL SYMPTOMS

This is a time when you may have some other strange sensations associated with menopause. All of them result from vasomotor instability and are considered to be hot-flash equivalents.

One of them is palpitations, which are distinct and rapid heartbeats. They are phenomena that are very common at menopause and do not signify heart trouble.

You may feel dizzy occasionally, or get faint now and then, or have a sensation similar to seasickness. Perhaps you get a strange salty or metallic sensation in your mouth. You have strange joint or muscle pains. Your eyes and perhaps your mouth feel dry. You feel irritable, tired, or weepy. You get headaches, are occasionally short of breath, or can't get to sleep at night.

You may notice peculiar sensations in your arms and hands, especially your fingers, and these too are vasomotor events. Some women describe them as tingling or pins and needles, while others get a feeling of numbness that comes and goes.

The strangest and often the most frightening menopausal symptom of all is formication, a crawling feeling over the skin. Luckily, this is rare. One patient thought these disquieting sensations signified an emotional breakdown and was greatly relieved to find out they were a typical menopausal occurrence. She was even more relieved to discover she could promptly banish her crawling skin with hormone replacement.

"Doctor, I Can't Sleep!"

Almost every woman suffers from insomnia, minor or major, when she becomes estrogen-deficient. Sometimes the problem lasts for years.

Some physicians think that sleeping problems are merely the result of hot flashes, with the heat and the sweating responsible for waking you up. It certainly is true that nobody can sleep through a severe hot flash that causes intense heat and so much perspiration that nightclothes and perhaps the sheets and even the mattress are soaked. Almost all hot flashes are associated with waking episodes.

But menopausal insomnia is more than that. First of all, women with an estrogen deficiency don't sleep as soundly as they once did. They spend less time in deep REM sleep and more time sleeping lightly and fitfully. They also experience changes in sleep patterns and brain waves from the same hypothalamic disturbances that cause hot flashes and an overstimulated central nervous system. A classic menopausal symptom is *sleep latency increase*, the inability to fall asleep after getting into bed and closing your eyes. Another is waking up in the middle of the night and tossing around for an hour or two. Between hot flashes and these disturbances, getting enough sleep can become a big problem.

Insomnia is second only to hot flashes as the reason why women make appointments to see their doctors during this time of physiological change.

All in Your Head?

If you tend to feel emotionally fragile around the time of menopause, don't be surprised. Among the symptoms commonly attributed to this absolutely normal phase of life are depression, irritability, fatigue, tension, instability, and anxiety. Although menopause won't make an emotionally healthy woman "go crazy" or cause major clinical depression, as people used to think, it definitely has an emotional component and it is not all in your head. There is a real and measurable physiological aspect to it.

Women have described their feelings as very similar to premenstrual syndrome (PMS). Although it has become unfashionable to blame any mood swings on "the change of life," estrogen *is* a mood-elevating hormone, and a drop in the amount circulating in your bloodstream *can* affect your emotions. So if you are feeling off-center, it may make you feel better to know it is not your imagination.

A shift in almost any hormone of any variety can affect mood and, in fact, psychological symptoms are often used in diagnosing hormonal imbalances. Estrogen is no exception. Just like the other variable symptoms, the periods of emotional stress occur most often and most noticeably in women whose hormone supply is abruptly or rapidly ended. They also correlate very closely with the fluctuations of hormone levels that occur over and over again during the climacteric.

Much Like PMS

Premenstrual syndrome has been shown to correlate with low levels of estrogen and high levels of progesterone just before the menstrual period. It's a time when many women feel irritable, edgy, and tense. Then, when their estrogen level rises again, their mood improves. Similar changes take place after the delivery of a baby. During pregnancy, the estrogen level rises about a thousand times. When the baby is born it plummets, frequently precipitating mood changes and depression.

In a less dramatic but equally valid biological way, your emotions respond to your decreasing estrogen level at menopause. This is a physiological response, although it may be exacerbated, of course, by psychological reactions to this tangible sign of growing older. If you consider menopause a discouraging symbol of approaching age, you will feel depressed at least temporarily, of course. But your feelings are also influenced by your physical state. If you keep that fact in mind and remember that this too will pass, you can distance yourself from it.

And it will probably pass quite quickly. The emotional component of menopause is an early symptom and almost always fades away in less than a year or two.

Strictly Psychological

Whatever emotional responses are triggered by hormonal changes often become intensified by our feelings about ourselves at this time of our lives. Few of us in this youth-oriented society can be expected to lose our major symbol of youthfulness—our fertility—and have no unhappy feelings about it. For almost everyone, menopause has its depressing and distressing aspects.

This is frequently a time for an identity crisis, a time to assess our accomplishments and abilities and to find them lacking. The arrival of menopause seems to focus attention on the negative aspects of our lives, the things we haven't done or been, the opportunities we have missed. It makes us fear we are becoming less attractive and sexually desirable.

But, in truth, menopause need not mean a loss of anything but menstrual periods and concern about getting pregnant. You can be just as feminine, interesting, and sexually able as you ever were, if not more so. As more women learn more about their bodies and refuse to accept the values and standards about menopause and middle age imposed on them by the social mythology, they discover that this is but one more chance to take stock of themselves and their lives—and to move on.

OTHER INTERESTING HAPPENINGS

Menopause is also the time for other physical changes that may make you wonder what is going on. These changes are not always directly related to low levels of estrogen but, because they tend to begin around the time of menopause, it is thought that there may be some link between them.

Weight Gain

Most women have a tendency to gain weight, sometimes as much as 10 pounds, in the first two to four years after menopause, even when their eating and exercise habits stay the same. Unfortunately, estrogen therapy may contribute to this tendency because it can promote water retention, although it does not cause weight gain per se. In fact, it has been found that women who take HRT tend to gain significantly less weight than those who don't. The problem is that this is the time of your life when your metabolism starts to slow down, your muscle mass decreases, and your body fat increases. Fat doesn't require as many calories to sustain it as muscle does. The only option you have is to cut back on your calorie intake and exercise more. To deal with the water retention, try cutting down on salt. Or take a diuretic occasionally, perhaps vitamin B_6, a natural diuretic, to help you with it.

Changing Shape

After menopause, the configuration of your body, the distribution of weight on your bones, begins to change. Hips and breasts tend to lose some of their fat tissue. Shoulders, upper back, and abdomen become thicker, while your waistline and rib cage expand and you may notice you've developed a little pot belly. You also lose height with the years and by age 50 you may be an inch or so shorter than you were when you were young. In the next few decades, you will lose more inches, perhaps two or three, as the spinal column compresses.

Hormone replacement therapy doesn't have much effect on weight distribution, although it may help somewhat to keep the pounds in their original locations. The best advice we can offer is to pare down your diet, especially the fats, and step up your exercise.

Suddenly Snoring

Many women start snoring after menopause and one of the reasons probably is that the mucous membranes in the nose (and in the mouth and eyes) become dryer, a direct result of a decreased supply of estrogen. Sometimes HRT will help.

Assorted Aches and Pains

Other common complaints around this time include backaches, especially in the pelvic area, and muscle pains. One reason for backaches is that one of estrogen's jobs is to help maintain the protein matrix of the spine and the density of the bones. Its absence may partially explain the aching and feelings of weakness.

The muscle pains probably reflect a reduction in muscular strength as a result of the drop in estrogen, along with a diminished ability to eliminate lactic acid after exercising.

Arthritic Pains

Joint pains, usually caused by osteoarthritis, also tend to begin or get worse around the time of menopause. We don't know if there is a direct connection between arthritic joint pains and an estrogen deficiency, but we do know that HRT will not make your condition worse and, in fact, it often dramatically relieves both muscle and joint pains after only about two weeks of treatment.

Dry Eyes

It is common for women to develop dry eyes after menopause because estrogen deficiency decreases the fluid production in many parts of the body, including the eyes, nose, mouth, and vagina. Artificial tears will help and so may HRT, as well as local application of sterile estrogen drops. Do not use decongestant eye drops because they can make your condition worse.

Dry Mouth

The decrease in estrogen that occurs at menopause can trigger dry mouth too, perhaps accompanied by strange taste sensations, sensitivity to hot and cold, and bleeding gums. If HRT doesn't help, try sucking sugarless candy to stimulate saliva.

COPING WITH THE SYMPTOMS

Hormone replacement therapy will promptly banish all of the transient symptoms of a changing estrogen level and, within a week or two, turn them into mere memories. But if your symptoms aren't very severe or you can't take estrogen because of previous battles with malignancies, there are some alternative measures that may work well enough to help you through. See the next chapter if you want to try them.

THE LONG-TERM MENOPAUSAL EFFECTS

Unlike hot flashes and the other temporary symptoms of menopause that go away as your body adjusts to your new estrogen deficiency, there are several *much* more important changes that occur in *all* women who don't take estrogen after menopause. These are atrophic tissue changes that develop gradually, always intensify with time, and remain with you forever unless you take HRT.

Every woman's timetable for these universal physical changes is different. They will appear much sooner if your menopause occurs abruptly than if your hormone supply diminishes slowly and you continue to make some estrogen in your ovaries and fat tissue. They include:

• Vaginal changes that can make sex extremely uncomfortable or even impossible and that encourage infections.

• Changes in the urethra that also invite discomfort and infections.

• The decreased ability of your bones to absorb and retain calcium, making them gradually become more brittle and breakable.

• The tendency for your beneficial HDL cholesterol level to decrease, your harmful LDL cholesterol to increase, and your arteries to accumulate plaque and become less elastic.

In addition to those important changes—direct results of estrogen deprivation—there are other events, major and minor, that happen sooner or later after menopause. For example, the bladder, another organ that is dependent on estrogen, loses muscle tone and elasticity, becoming less able to hold urine. The muscles of the pelvic floor become lax. The breasts lose their thick layer of fat and the milk glands shrink. The skin too loses its underlying layer of fat and becomes thinner, dryer, and less resilient.

Most women, if they choose, can manage to live through the variable transient symptoms of menopause without medical help because the symptoms will eventually subside whatever they do. But the universal physical changes will never fade away with time and, in fact, they get progressively worse, sometimes dramatically affecting the quality of life. With HRT, however, all of them are arrested, ameliorated, or reversed.

After a discussion in the next chapter of the alternative treatments for hot flashes and the other vasomotor symptoms, we are going to talk about the three major universal changes one by one.

In Chapter 8, we will discuss the effects of menopause on your vagina and, therefore, your sex life—and what you can do about them.

Chapter 9 focuses on changes in the tissues that encourage vaginal and urinary infections.

Chapter 10 is about your bones, your chances of developing symptomatic osteoporosis, and how you can prevent it.

6

HRT or Not: The Alternative Therapies

••

If you wait long enough, your hot flashes, insomnia, crawly skin, and other strange menopausal symptoms will all go away. Time is the cure. If you are one of the lucky ones whom they don't bother very much, just wait them out. But if you've got symptoms that make you miserable, especially if they last for years, fight back! Refuse to accept them! Take charge of your own life!

HRT is the only good answer for women whose bones, hearts, or sex lives are in danger. But, if your only concern is uncomfortable symptoms, try the nondrug remedies described in this chapter before resorting to any medication, including hormone replacement therapy.

If the alternative measures don't help you enough, however, remember that replacing the hormones your body no longer makes will not endanger your health, no matter what you've seen on television or heard from friends and relations, if you use it correctly and follow your doctor's orders.

NATURAL REMEDIES

For menopausal symptoms that are not too bothersome, try these natural remedies.

Vitamin E

Vitamin E often does a commendable job of relieving the severity and frequency of flashes and other symptoms. Start with 400 units of vitamin E twice a day (800 total). If that doesn't work, double the dose for a daily total of 1,600 units.

Nobody really knows exactly how vitamin E works because, unlike the other vitamins, it is not manufactured by the human body and must be provided by foods and supplements. But it produces remarkable results for many women whose symptoms are not overwhelming.

It's always best to get vitamins from your diet if you can manage it, because supplements usually do not contain all of the nutritional components found in foods. The richest dietary sources of vitamin E are vegetable oils, nuts, and whole grains, with wheat germ oil by far the richest source. Keep in mind that much of the vitamin is lost in cooking, processing, and storage.

In the case of vitamin E, you can't possibly get anywhere near as much as you need for relieving menopausal symptoms if you rely on food sources alone. Most dietary sources of vitamin E are rich in oils so also high in fat and calories. To get the vitamin E contained in a typical 400 IU supplement capsule, you would have to eat a pound of sunflower seeds or two quarts of corn oil, the equivalent of about 8,000 calories a day. That means you must get this vitamin in the form of supplements.

B-Complex and Vitamin C

There has also been testimony, although no scientific studies to back it up, that the B vitamins and vitamin C can help relieve menopausal symptoms. Try increasing your intakes of both B-complex and C. They certainly won't do you any harm if you don't overdo them and they may do you some good. Start with one B-50 tablet,

400 to 500 mg of vitamin B$_6$, and 500 mg of C once a day and see if you get relief.

Good Nutrition

Nutrition plays an important role in estrogen production, so it is important to be sure your diet is sensible, well balanced, and adequate. Women who exist on extreme low-protein diets often have such decreased hormone production that they fail to ovulate or have menstrual periods.

So do women who exist for a good portion of their lives on subnormal numbers of calories. It is *impossible* to get adequate nutrition on less than about 1,200 calories a day. Low-calorie diets are unhealthy if you stay on them longer than a week or two. So are high-protein diets, which contribute to the risk of developing osteoporosis.

Fruits and Vegetables

Cut back on animal products and eat more plant foods and you may find your symptoms alleviated. Naturally occurring plant estrogens (phytoestrogens) are found in many plant foods such as apples, alfalfa sprouts, split peas, spinach, and especially soybean products. The phytoestrogens compete with more powerful human estrogens in binding to the body's estrogen receptors, according to Cornell University researchers.

Ginseng

Ginseng, a root that's been used for centuries as a folk medicine to relieve flashes and other "women's troubles," happens to be a potent source of plant estrogen, as are several other plant materials.

If you take it for hot flashes and other symptoms, you are now taking estrogen replacement therapy. Ginseng may be a "natural" estrogen, but it is still estrogen and has the same effects on your body as taking the hormone in pills, patches, or creams. Furthermore, you are getting it unopposed by progesterone, and so you may build up excessive amounts of uterine lining and develop hyperplasia if you use it continually and/or in high doses. Because you have no way of knowing how much phytoestrogen you are getting with ginseng, you will never know if you are overdosing.

So, if you are going to take it to relieve symptoms, do it sparingly, always keeping in mind that you are actually taking estrogen without the important protection of progesterone.

MORE NATURAL REMEDIES

There are other estrogenlike plant materials—for example, dong quai, wild yam, evening primrose oil, sage, chamomile, catnip, hops, passionflower, and wild turnips—that women swear have helped them cope with symptoms. Again, the amount of estrogen they provide is a mystery. And, because they have not yet been the subjects of controlled studies or adequately tested for safety, it is impossible to evaluate them objectively. But taken *in moderation*, these herbs with estrogenlike effects won't be harmful and they may be helpful if your symptoms are mild. On the other hand, heavy and prolonged use of plant estrogens can cause hyperplasia, an overproliferation of the endometrium, which can lead to uterine cancer.

Another remedy that has gained popularity recently is Pro-gest cream or oil applied on the abdomen and buttocks. Pro-gest contains progesterone synthesized from Mexican yams and its purpose is to relieve many female complaints, including menopausal symptoms. If you try it, remember that it is not known how much of this substance is absorbed into the bloodstream and exactly how it will perform.

Dong Quai

This herb acts like an estrogen, although it does not cause hyperplasia, and it can alleviate hot flashes for some women. It is not recommended, however, because it contains psoralen, a known carcinogen, as well as an anticoagulant that can be dangerous.

Black Cohash

To date, black cohash taken for menopausal symptoms seems to be safe and is approved in Germany for a maximum of six months for dysmenorrhea (menstrual pain). It can lower blood pressure, however, and for some people that is not desirable.

Promensil (Red Clover)

An isoflavone or plant estrogen derived from red clover, Promensil, now sold over-the-counter in the United States, has been extensively studied in Australia where it has been marketed for many years. In our 1998–1999 study of this drug at New York University Medical Center, we found that this product significantly reduced the number of hot flashes for most women, even for one volunteer who had been suffering from more than 40 flashes a day. It always decreased their intensity and often stopped them completely after about four weeks.

Australian research has shown that Promensil may improve bone density and protect against both heart disease and breast cancer, but this work has not yet been duplicated in the United States. We do know from our own work, however, that short-term use of 40 mg daily does not increase endometrial thickness.

Soy Products

Soy is a weak plant estrogen that, for some women, seems to reduce the severity of menopausal symptoms such as hot flashes. And there is some evidence, mostly anecdotal, that a diet rich in soy products can reduce the risk factors for cardiovasular disease and osteoporosis among postmenopausal women. Other claims have been made that it can lower LDL cholesterol and offer protection against breast cancer, but there has been no scientific research to back them up. Nor is there any proof that Chinese or Japanese women have a lower incidence of breast cancer because they eat a lot of soy.

Meanwhile, adding soy to your diet won't hurt you and it may be beneficial since it is a good low-fat source of protein. On the other hand, the quantity required to be effective for hot flashes means you must take in enormous amounts of fat and calories. Soy supplements are not yet subject to regulation or quality control, so their purity and dosage are uncertain. Watch for a new concentrated soy product, however, that eliminates the fat.

Natural, Yes, But Are They Safe?

"Natural" is not synonymous with "safe." Although most herbal remedies are not dangerous, at least in the short run and in small doses, they must be used with caution. Keep in mind that they are not always good for you. Despite new research, women with a history of breast or uterine cancer shouldn't take any additional estrogen—including plant-based estrogen—without first consulting their doctor.

Remember too that it is possible—and quite common—to overdose on herbs and other natural products that have an effect on body functions. If you do, you may get some unexpected and unwelcome reactions. Some can cause allergic reactions, while others can be toxic and hazardous when consumed in large quantities. Always buy them at a reputable store and ask for the recommended dosage.

Keep in mind, too, that these "dietary supplements" or

nutrients have not been tested, regulated, or approved by the FDA or any other regulatory agency. That means manufacturers are not required to test them for safety. Nor must they guarantee that they are pure, contain what the label claims they do, or provide uniform doses. The products contained in them are not subject to pre-market government regulation and may be adulterated, especially if the active ingredient is very expensive or hard to obtain. Furthermore, there are no rules governing recommended dosages.

A report published in early 1995 in the *Journal of the American Medical Association* described a case of severe liver and kidney damage resulting from daily doses of chaparral, an herbal compound made from a desert shrub. The report elicited warnings that many herbal products are toxic to human livers.

Rejuvex, marketed vigorously today, is another story because it does not come from plants but instead is made of "glandular powders" derived from "bovine sources," with some vitamins added to the mix. Better to take your vitamins straight.

TELL YOUR DOCTOR

Herbal remedies can cause adverse reactions that can be undiagnosed and mistreated if your doctor doesn't know what you're taking. Some herbs aggravate chronic conditions such as diabetes, arthritis, and hypertension, or interact harmfully with other medications. Large doses of garlic, for example, could interact dangerously with anticoagulants. Ginseng may lower blood sugar excessively for diabetics on medication. Therefore, it is very important to consult with your physician before you start taking herbal supplements and again when any new drugs are prescribed.

ACUPUNCTURE, BIOFEEDBACK, RELAXATION TECHNIQUES

Some women have reported that acupuncture can help relieve the severity and frequency of flashes and, in fact, both acupuncture and biofeedback are currently under study to determine their real effects on menopausal symptoms.

Deep abdominal breathing can reduce the frequency of hot flashes, according one study, so why not give it a try? Morning and night, breathe slowly and deeply—six to eight times a minute—for about 10 minutes.

You may also want to try relaxation techniques such as visualization and meditation, which have been found to ease many kinds of discomforts and will certainly help you cope with the stress they can cause.

VIGOROUS EXERCISE

Always a good idea, sufficient vigorous exercise may be another way to ease your way through menopause. According to a study at the University of Illinois, women who spend the most time dancing or playing tennis experience fewer hot flashes, night sweats, and mood swings.

SENSIBLE SOLUTIONS

Do whatever you can to cool off when flashes and sweats overtake you. Avoid hot drinks, caffeine, spicy foods, and alcohol. Have a cold drink or a cool shower. They'll help you feel better for the moment. So will air-conditioning, layered clothes that you can peel off, cool weather, low humidity, sufficient rest, peace, and serenity. Try them.

MEDICAL ALTERNATIVES TO ESTROGEN

There is nothing that can relieve symptoms as effectively as estrogen. It works for 98 percent of its users—and it works fast. Within a week to 10 days on a minimal dose, flashes and the other vasomotor phenomena are events of the past.

But if you must avoid estrogen, there are a few alternative medical treatments. They don't work as well as HRT but, for some women, they provide relief. We list them here.

Progesterone

Progesterone, the second most important female hormone, may be prescribed alone, without estrogen, to help decrease the frequency and severity of flashes and the other transient vasomotor events. Although it is nowhere near as effective as estrogen, 2.5 mg of oral medroxyprogesterone a day can sometimes be helpful when nothing else works. Ask your doctor about taking megestrol acetate (Megace), the only kind of progesterone that's been approved by the FDA for women who have had breast cancer. Low doses of this drug were found in a study at the Mayo Clinic to reduce the frequency of hot flashes by an average of 85 percent among women who couldn't take estrogen.

Another choice is Depo-Provera, a long-acting progesterone that works exceptionally well at banishing the symptoms. Approved as a contraceptive by the FDA, it is injected intramuscularly every three months in doses of 150 mg. If your doctor will administer it, your troubles may be over.

Tranquilizers and Sedatives

Tranquilizers, especially those like Valium that suppress hypothalamic function, are another medical method of diminishing symptoms. Although they should not be used for long periods of time because they are habit-forming and your body tends to build up a tolerance to them, they sometimes work well. So do sedatives, which accomplish the same goal by decreasing autonomic nervous system irritability. But use them cautiously and only temporarily because they are potentially addictive.

Clonidine

Clonidine (Catapres), a drug normally used for hypertension, sometimes provides some relief from flashes. If you can't take estrogen, this is probably your next best choice after progesterone. A problem is that it may lower normal blood pressure.

Lofexidine

This is an alpha-blocker that can significantly decrease vasomotor episodes and may be helpful when estrogen therapy is out of the question. Problem: It too lowers blood pressure and sometimes decreases libido.

Bellergal-S

An antispasmodic drug that occasionally diminishes hot flashes, Bellergal is not commonly recommended because of its possible side effects such as a slowdown of digestion and blurred vision. A compound containing phenobarbital and belladonna, it should be among your last options if estrogen is ruled out.

Tibolone

A drug that is used in many other countries and is currently undergoing clinical trials in the United States, tibolone (marketed as Liviol) has estrogenlike effects on flashes, vaginal dryness, bones, and heart, but does not cause hyperplasia, the excessive proliferation of the endometrium, or increased breast activity. Therefore, it is a drug with great future promise for women who have had breast cancer.

GETTING A GOOD NIGHT'S SLEEP

All the transient menopausal symptoms, including insomnia, usually vanish within a few days after starting estrogen replacement therapy.

But if your symptoms don't seem severe enough to warrant hormone treatment, or you don't choose to go that route, there are other ways to travel in your search for a good night's sleep. The usual remedies well known to insomniacs apply here too. It is important to remember that, in most cases, your sleeping problems are temporary, probably won't occur every night, and will improve with time.

The over-the-counter sleep medications, usually mild antihistamines, have some sleep-inducing properties and may help you if you use them only occasionally. But try to stay away from prescription sleep-inducers because they have a dangerous overdose potential and can become addictive. Besides, they reduce the REM or deep stage of sleep and lose their effectiveness after a while.

Again, it's best to try the natural remedies before resorting to medications. One is warm milk, which contains tryptophan, an amino acid that acts as a sedative. So do certain other foods such as tuna fish. A tuna fish sandwich and a glass of warm milk may be all you need to put you to sleep for the night. Stay away, however, from tryptophan supplements because an overdose can be dangerous and can cause eosinophilic granuloma, an arthritic condition.

Other natural sleep-inducers that work for many people include wine (a small amount only, or it may have the opposite effect in the middle of the night), warm (not

hot) baths, exercise (not too close to bedtime), ginseng
and herbal teas, vitamin B-complex, calcium, and vitamin
C. Check them out.

Small doses of the natural hormone melatonin may
work too, although this hormone is still under study and
has an overdose potential. Start out with a dose of 1 mg
every night before you go to bed. Sometimes even half of
that does the job, though some women need more. Take
it every night because the effect is cumulative.

The experts on insomnia say that you probably get
enough sleep despite your waking episodes, and that the
less you worry about it the better. Just remember that the
remedy that always works is time. When your body
adjusts to its new low levels of hormones, you will sleep
again.

COPING WITH MOOD SWINGS

Time is once again your best friend. Keep in mind that
your physiologically induced mood swings will level out
eventually. An early menopausal symptom, they rarely
last longer than a year. If you decide to start hormone
therapy, they will improve within a week or so.

In the meantime, you may want to join the many other
women who use nutritional methods of achieving better
emotional equilibrium. Although there has been no scientific verification of its effectiveness, many people think
that taking vitamin B-complex (the "antistress vitamin")
is helpful. You can get B vitamins in foods such as liver
and whole grains and you can also get them in supplements. Try taking a B-complex tablet (50 or 100 mg) every
day.

Calcium is also recommended by nutritionists for emotional stress (you should be consuming considerable
amounts of it now in any case to help fight osteoporosis),
and vitamin C has its supporters, who extol it for its

calming effect. So does vitamin E, as well as all the sooth-
ing herbal teas. If these natural remedies work for you,
they may help you avoid drugs.

Obviously, if your emotional state is primarily due to
your changing hormone level, then hormone replacement therapy can provide dramatic relief. Estrogen,
which affects the central nervous system, can improve
mood and feelings of well-being. If it works for you—
remember it may be used only temporarily—you can
avoid other more powerful drugs. If it is not medically
contraindicated in your case, try it before you get into
tranquilizers or antidepressants. Taking HRT under a
qualified physician's supervision, if only for the year or
two it takes for the symptoms to subside, is not only safe
but sane.

The tranquilizers such as Valium that suppress the
hypothalamus are frequently recommended for emotional stress at menopause. They have a sedative and
muscle-relaxing effect and can help you sleep too.
Antidepressants are also frequently prescribed and can
work wonders for the blues, whatever their source. If all
else has failed, and you can't take estrogen, ask your doctor about prescribing them for you. They are not harmful
if you use them correctly, cautiously, and temporarily.

7

HORMONE REPLACEMENT THERAPY: WHAT, WHEN, HOW, WHY

••

Estrogen can work wonders, producing results no other drug can accomplish anywhere near as well, but like all drugs, it must be used correctly. In this chapter we give you the latest, most up-to-the-minute word on HRT, what it does and doesn't do for you, and how to use it safely.

Here is where you will get all the information you need about the logistics of hormone replacement: how you and your doctor will know if you need it, how to take it, and the three alternate ways to use it—the pills, the patches, and the creams. You will learn about dosages, precautions, possible side effects, contraindications, and the right way to quit if that's what you decide to do.

MAKING A DECISION ABOUT ESTROGEN

If your symptoms and physical changes aren't too severe and you are *not* a prime candidate for osteoporosis or early heart disease, some of the nondrug alternatives we have described may work well enough to get you by. If they don't help you enough, however, don't let your fears or your friends talk you out of hormone therapy. It is safe and effective if you do it *right*. Every woman should seriously consider taking HRT after menopause if she has no medical contraindications because, for virtually all women, the benefits, especially for their bones, their hearts, and their vaginas, far outweigh the risks.

Taking hormones is not a lifetime commitment. You can stop whenever you like. You may decide you don't need HRT anymore or you may decide that you don't want to take it anymore. If you want it only to relieve symptoms, then two to five years should be enough. For sexual problems, you need it as long as you are sexually active. To prevent osteoporosis, you should stay on HRT for life. But you don't have to decide *now* how long you'll stay on it. Wait for your next gynecological checkup to decide how you feel about it and what you want to do.

WHAT YOU SHOULD KNOW ABOUT HRT

Before making a decision about taking hormone replacement therapy, consider the following facts.

• Some women never need HRT. Others can manage to get along without it if they choose to or they must.

• Some women shouldn't take it, just as there are women who shouldn't take aspirin or penicillin. Today, however, this group is almost exclusively limited to women who have had estrogen-dependent cancer.

• There are women who require estrogen for the short term only, just long enough to get through their hot flashes and other uncomfortable symptoms. HRT is considered short term when it is taken for anywhere from a few months to five years. With rare exceptions, all women can safely take short-term therapy.

• Many women need estrogen for many years or for the rest of their lives. These are the women who are especially susceptible to developing symptomatic osteoporosis, brittle bones that are subject to disabling or even life-threatening fractures, or are likely to get coronary heart disease. Nothing works as well as estrogen to prevent or arrest osteoporosis. Nothing works as well as estrogen for lowering dangerous cholesterol levels or keeping arteries elastic. And nothing works as well as estrogen for alleviating persistent vaginal and urethral infections, and preventing vaginal changes that can turn you off to sex.

• Women who are prime candidates for osteoporosis should not waste valuable time. They *must* take estrogen promptly after menopause to prevent the irreversible bone loss that begins at that time. If they cannot take HRT, they must monitor their bone density and use one of the new alternatives described in Chapter 10.

• Women who are prime candidates for coronary artery disease and heart attacks should not waste a lot of time either. If you have a family history of heart disease, especially among the female members of the family, this means you. It also means you if you already have symptoms of heart disease, or if your HDL cholesterol level drops markedly soon after menopause.

• HRT is not the same as oral contraception. The pill adds hormones to a woman's already normal hormone level. The hormones in HRT replace the hormones you no longer make for yourself and never give you anywhere near the amount you once produced from your own ovaries or the dose you would get from most contraceptives. The usual daily dose of 0.625 mg of conjugated estrogen (or the equivalent dose of other estrogen) is only about one-fourth of the amount in the newest very-low-dose birth control pills. And, incidentally, it is only a quarter of what was routinely prescribed for post-menopausal women a couple of decades ago.

• Occasionally, HRT has side effects, most of them minor and temporary, such as water retention and nausea. If they are too uncomfortable or become hazardous, you can quit the hormones and they will disappear.

• Estrogen, like any other drug, should not be taken casually. It must be individualized specifically for you and then monitored regularly. It should be "opposed" by progesterone if you have a uterus. And it should be taken in the smallest amount that will accomplish its purpose.

WHO CAN'T TAKE IT?

Hormone replacement therapy is safe for virtually every postmenopausal woman today *except* those who have had estrogen-dependent breast cancer, recent advanced endometrial cancer, or currently have acute and active liver disease or active thrombophlebitis.

And there are exceptions even to this general rule: Oncologists occasionally approve vaginal estrogen cream today to relieve severe vaginal or urinary problems in breast cancer patients who have been free of the disease for several years. A panel of experts recently reviewed 24 studies of the possible connection between estrogen and breast cancer and concluded that it is very doubtful that the hormone causes cancer, although it can accelerate the growth of cancer cells that are *already* present. And a study reported in 1994 in the *Journal of the American*

Medical Association found no evidence that HRT could reactivate dormant cancer cells. It is now considered safe even for breast cancer patients when it is taken for less than three years.

Until very recently, estrogen was also denied to women who once had uterine cancer but, according to the newest thinking among gynecologic oncologists, the benefits generally outweigh the risks of stimulating leftover cancer cells to grow. So it is now usually considered permissable to take it unless the cancer was advanced or occurred within the last year.

Because estrogen can make very large fibroids grow even larger, these benign muscle tumors may be another contraindication to HRT, but not always. Fibroids are not initiated by estrogen, but they depend on it for their growth, growing fastest in the years of plentiful hormones and shrinking after menopause. Deciding whether you should take HRT if you have potentially troublesome fibroids is a matter of judgment, but it is always possible to try the hormones and see what effect they have. Or to wait a few years until the fibroids have shrunk before starting replacement therapy. HRT, because it contains such a low dose of estrogen, rarely makes fibroids grow.

Not too many years ago, women were advised not to take long-term hormone replacement if they had certain preexisting medical conditions such as liver impairment, gallbladder disease, a specific type of hypertension, or thrombophlebitis. Today, however, you can take it safely even with those problems if you use the transdermal patch or vaginal cream. Both the patch and the cream deliver estrogen through the skin directly into the bloodstream without alteration by the digestive system and, as a result, they are safe for you. For more discussion, see Chapter 2.

HOW HORMONE REPLACEMENT WORKS

Ideally, estrogen should be taken in a physiologic way, matching as closely as possible the normal premenopausal pattern of a steady amount of estrogen throughout the month overlapped by progesterone for 10 to 14 days.

Oral estrogen has traditionally been prescribed three weeks of the month with one week off simply because physicians have copied the schedule devised for birth control pills when a week off was required to allow for a menstrual period. But today it is considered best to take it every day of the month because this pattern provides a constant level of the hormone circulating in the bloodstream and affords better protection for the bones and heart. It also averts the mood swings and PMS-like feelings that are common during the "week off."

For several reasons that we will soon discuss, you may choose to take progesterone every day of the month too. Given in very small daily doses, it adds up to about the same amount as taking the customary larger daily doses for only 10 or 12 or 14 days a month and does not affect the beneficial effect of estrogen on your cholesterol level or bone density.

PERIODS AGAIN?

Every month, if you take progesterone cyclically, you may have a brief period or "menstrual response." This doesn't signify a return to fertility but simply means the progesterone is doing its job of cleaning out the uterus after the estrogen builds it up. The progesterone changes the cells of the lining from proliferative to secretory. When you stop taking it after its allotted number of days, the secretions carry out all the accumulated blood and proliferated cells, leaving the endometrium clean and healthy right down to the basement membrane, just as it should be.

If you take progesterone cyclically each month and don't get a short menstrual period in response, there's no reason to be concerned. That's even better than having the period because it means the estrogen is not causing the endometrium to build up each month and so there is no excessive material to clear out. But period or not, you must continue to take the progesterone as long as you take the estrogen if you have not had a hysterectomy.

If you get periods with progesterone, they should be lighter and shorter than your former menstrual periods. In most cases, they last only a couple of days and produce only a very light or moderate flow. You will probably have them once a month for about 8 to 10 years and then they will stop forever.

Periods Are Not Popular

The reappearance of menstrual periods, even these abbreviated responses, are seldom greeted with enthusiasm and they are the most common complaint women have about taking hormones. In fact, they are probably the most usual reason given for not choosing to start the therapy or for quitting it later on.

But, like them or not, progesterone is *essential* if you haven't had a hysterectomy and therefore have a uterus, and you should not stop taking it unless you quit the estrogen too. Progesterone is what makes HRT so safe today.

Avoiding the Periods

There is a way, however, to take progesterone and yet avoid having periods. If you dislike having periods so much that you are contemplating quitting hormone therapy because of them, ask your gynecologist to prescribe the progesterone in very low doses in a continuous *everyday* pattern. This means you take estrogen every day, by pill or patch, *and* a low dose (2.5 mg or 5 mg) of medroxyprogesterone acetate (Provera) or an equivalent dose of other progesterone every day. For 8 out of every 10 women, this regime puts an end to the periods. Typically, you'll have minor periods or spotting for the first two or three months and then none at all.

If you are among the 20 percent of women who continue to have irregular or heavy bleeding on the new regime, however, then you must go back to the cyclical schedule.

Taking progesterone continuously seems to be just as safe as taking it cyclically and it does not alter the beneficial effects of estrogen on raising your HDLs, the "good" cholesterol, and maintaining the elasticity of your arteries.

PROGESTERONE'S SIDE EFFECTS

For some women, progesterone is a downer. It makes them jumpy, tense, anxious, depressed. In fact, it feels like PMS, which is also caused by a rise in the blood level of progesterone. These feelings are usually temporary, fading away about three months after you start HRT. But if they are persistent, try taking your progesterone in very low doses in the continuous every-day-of-the-month pattern described above and see if you can tolerate it then. Under your gynecologist's supervision, try different regimes to arrive at the dose that's comfortable for you. Whatever works is fine, as long as your endometrium remains perfectly normal.

Another route to try if you can't take progesterone by mouth is by suppository. Suppositories can be made up to order by your pharmacist at the direction of your gynecologist.

If nothing helps and you absolutely cannot tolerate

progesterone's side effects, you can safely quit taking it. But *only* if you follow certain rigid rules.

Here are the rules. First, there must be no "break-through" or unscheduled vaginal bleeding because that means your endometrium has been overstimulated on estrogen alone. Second, you must have an endometrial biopsy to test for hyperplasia, once a year at first; then if all goes well, every other year. Or, as an alternative, you must have an ultrasound examination to measure the thickness of your uterine lining. If the endometrium is less than 6 mm thick, then we know you have not developed hyperplasia.

"NATURAL" PROGESTERONES

Synthetic progesterones known as progestins—medroxy-progesterone acetate (Provera) and norethindrone acetate (Aygestin)—are made from plants but chemically altered so they can be better absorbed by the body. The only forms of progesterone on the market for many years, they now have competition from a couple of "natural" alternatives.

One, called Prometrium, is a capsule containing yam-derived micronized progesterone in peanut oil. Prometrium was approved by the FDA in 1998 for treating amenor-rhea (absence of periods) but is now used for HRT as well. Advantages include less fluid retention and less effect on HDL cholesterol levels. Its major side effect is that it makes you very sleepy, so be sure to take it at night. Although it is not quite as effective at cleaning out the uterine lining as the synthetic progestins, Prometrium is not only natural but seems to have fewer unpleasant side effects.

So now you have another option and another decision to make. Prometrium comes in 100 mg capsules that can be taken along with estrogen every day of the month if you have chosen the continuous schedule. On a cyclic schedule, you would require three of the 100 mg capsules per day for 10 to 12 days a month overlapping your daily estrogen.

Crinone, a prescription vaginal gel made from yams, is another natural FDA-approved micronized progesterone product. It is applied locally in the vagina with premeasured prefilled applicators to be absorbed through the mucous membranes and the lymphatic system directly into the lining of the uterus, where it protects it from hyperplasia. Crinone is a boon for women who can't tolerate oral progesterone. Because very little is absorbed into the general circulation when used in a 4 percent dose, it rarely causes any of the typical unpleasant side effects.

THE CYCLICAL PERIODS: WHAT TO EXPECT

When you take progesterone cyclically, you will probably have a short menstrual period six or more hours after your last dose of the month. It will be short (two to five days), unclotted, and light. It will follow the same pattern every month, varying no more than one or two days, and varying only slightly in the amount of flow. If, for example, you take progesterone from the first to the tenth day of the month and get a light menstrual response on the eleventh day, you should *always* get it on the eleventh (give or take a day or two) every single month and the flow should always be light.

If there is *any* other variation—in timing or flow—consider it abnormal bleeding and promptly check it out with your doctor. Heavy bleeding, for example, is never normal on HRT.

Sometimes you will bleed one month but not the next. If you don't bleed when you take progesterone, fine! It means your endometrium is in good shape.

Bleeding: Normal or Not?

The *only* vaginal bleeding now allowed is the menstrual response described above, always in the same pattern. If there is *any* bleeding at *any* time other than those usual few days, it must be investigated. It is abnormal. If the menstrual response to the progesterone lasts longer, if it contains clots, or it becomes heavy, you must promptly bring it to the attention of your physician. It could be caused by polyps in the cervix or uterus. It could come from fibroids. It could be hyperplasia or even early cancer. Whatever it is, your job is to check it out immediately.

In other words, *any bleeding that is not according to plan must be investigated.* Unscheduled bleeding is a warning sign, so always pay attention to it. Make an appointment with your gynecologist immediately for a complete pelvic examination that includes careful scrutiny of the endometrial cells under a microscope at a reputable laboratory.

Although the unscheduled bleeding rarely signifies a serious problem, time is important. If the doctor's office tries to put off your appointment more than two weeks, insist that you are given an earlier one.

Periods Are Not Forever

Your new periods, if you have them, will not continue forever. They will stop after a few years when the endometrium becomes nonfunctional and inactive, unable to build up that thickened lining that must be eliminated.

When this happens, continue taking your progesterone *as long as you take estrogen* and don't worry. Easy to say, but many women get a little apprehensive when the periods disappear, wondering if something is wrong. But this state of affairs is perfectly normal. It simply means you now have an inactive endometrium and there is nothing to clear out each month anymore.

THE PILL AS AN ALTERNATIVE

Although hormone replacement therapy before menopause is not recommended except in tiny amounts or
under certain circumstances, it is safe to use the new
very-low-dose birth control pills to relieve hot flashes
and other symptoms when they make an early appearance. The pills, approved by the FDA for women up to
the age of 50, contain estrogen as well as progesterone
and will accomplish four purposes. They will relieve the
menopausal symptoms, regulate your erratic periods,
stop dysfunctional bleeding, and prevent pregnancy all
at the same time. See Chapter 3 for more about the pill.

CAN YOU GET PREGNANT?

Once you are certifiably menopausal, you are no longer
fertile and you can't get pregnant despite the menstrual
responses to the progesterone.

But be sure to use contraception for at least a year after
your last real period, whether or not you take HRT, just
in case your ovaries decide to turn out one more viable
egg. Many a woman age 45 or 50 has been mighty surprised by this unsettling turn of events, and most of the
time it has not been a welcome surprise.

NO HRT BEFORE MENOPAUSE

As we have already explained, taking hormone replacement therapy before menopause is not recommended
except under special circumstances. In fact, it can be dangerous during the erratic periods of perimenopause
because that is a time when you may sometimes produce
huge peaks of estrogen in response to the frantic activities
of the pituitary gland to get your ovaries back in business.
If you are still having periods, however irregular, it means
you are still making enough estrogen to build up your

uterine lining. But because you are not ovulating regularly or at all, you are probably not producing the progesterone needed to eliminate that lining every month.

Exception: If you have severe menopausal symptoms that start while you are still having menstrual periods, your physician can examine the vaginal cells under a microscope. If no cornified cells (the cells that form a protective outer layer of the vaginal lining) are seen, your estrogen level is probably very low. In this special instance only, a brief course of HRT may be safely prescribed to relieve the symptoms.

Another exception: As we explained in Chapter 3, it is safe to take very tiny amounts of estrogen if you badly need them to alleviate severe symptoms. Climara is a skin patch that delivers only 0.025 mg of estrogen a day, giving you enough to relieve the symptoms without causing problems.

In any case, severe symptoms rarely make a grand entrance before your periods have gone for good. But if they do, talk to your doctor about taking very-low-dose birth control pills.

TESTING FOR MENOPAUSE

As a general rule, your estrogen level must be low and you must have had menopause before starting HRT. The best test for determining whether your ovarian function has diminished sufficiently, you are producing very little estrogen, and have had menopause, is a test of your FSH serum level. FSH, the follicle-stimulating hormone produced by the pituitary gland, is normally below 10 MIU/ml during your fertile years. The closer it gets to 40 MIU/ml, the closer you are to menopause. When it soars above that number, it's all over. You are making very little estrogen, no progesterone at all, and your ovaries have gone into retirement. Once the FSH level goes up, it usually stays up, perhaps for the rest of your life.

Although there are other methods of determining whether you are certifiably menopausal or are about to reach it, this is the most definitive test. Measurements of your circulating estrogen level may come up with misleading information, because that level may change from day to day, rising and falling unpredictably in response to the demands of your pituitary gland. Cervical smears rated according to the amount of estrogen present can provide only a rough indication of your status, but are not reliable because they do not measure your circulating estrogen. Observation of the vagina and cervix and the presence of obvious symptoms provide clues, of course, but do not always tell the real story.

So, if you want to know whether you have had menopause, have an FSH test.

STARTING HRT: THE PRELIMINARY STEPS

When you know you have reached menopause and have decided you want to start HRT, what happens next? These are the important preliminary procedures to be performed by your physician:

- A thorough physical examination, including a pelvic exam and a breast exam.

- A Pap smear.

- Complete blood tests for glucose level, liver function, thyroid and parathyroid function, cholesterol/triglyceride levels, calcium and phosphorus levels.

- Endometrial biopsy for close microscopic examination of the cells of the lining. Subsequently, your physician may use the progesterone challenge test or an ultrasound examination to rule out hyperplasia or cancer. See Chapter 13 for more about these options.

• Mammography (see Chapter 2).

• A complete family history, with special emphasis on osteoporosis, heart disease, and cancer.

• Bone-density tests for osteoporosis, if deemed necessary.

FOLLOW-UP VISITS

You should see your doctor about three months after you begin HRT to be sure you are doing it right. You'd be surprised, for example, how many women reverse their estrogen and progesterone doses. This will be an opportunity too for the physician to individualize your treatment. Every woman's response to hormones is different and not everyone responds the same way to the usual dosages, schedules, types of hormones, and routes of administration. The doctor can try different alternatives until one is found that is right for you.

The checkup visit is also another chance to ask questions. Few women get everything straight the first time around and, even if they do, most of them are afraid they haven't. Don't be afraid to ask questions, no matter how trivial or embarrassing they seem to you, and make sure you get satisfactory answers before leaving the office.

After that, you should schedule follow-up visits every six months.

TAKING HORMONES: THE ALTERNATIVES

There are several ways of taking hormones to replace those you no longer adequately produce on your own: pills, patches, creams, and rings. Each has its advantages and disadvantages and sometimes you have to try a couple of them before deciding which is best for you.

Oral Estrogen

Until recently, the only way to take estrogen replacement was by pill and it is still the way most women take it. Premarin, oral conjugated estrogen (a blend of naturally occurring estrogens) distilled from the urine of pregnant mares, has been available since 1941 and it is one of the most extensively tested medications in history. It is the most commonly prescribed estrogen replacement. And it is also the number one prescribed drug in the United States.

But there are many other choices of oral estrogens today, any one of which your doctor may prescribe for you. All of them have benefits thought to be similar to Premarin's. These include synthetic conjugated estrogens, pure estradiol from plant materials, synthetic and semisynthetic compounds, and a micronized form of natural estradiol. Among those derived from plants are Cenestin, Estrace, Estratab, and Menest, with more in the works. Others—Ogen and Ortho-Est—are synthesized from estrone.

Combination Pill

Now you don't have to take two pills every day or even part of the month to get both of your hormones. You can take just one, a combination of estrogen and progesterone in a single tablet, sold in dispensers containing a 28-day supply.

The combination pills come in two versions. Prempro provides daily doses of 0.625 mg of conjugated estrogen and 2.5 mg of progesterone. It is designed for women who take both hormones every day of the month. Premphase gives you the same number of tablets, but 14 of them contain daily doses of 0.625 mg of estrogen, while the other 14 contain daily doses of 0.625 mg of estrogen combined with 5 mg of progesterone. These are for women who do better with a cyclical progesterone schedule.

Transdermal Estrogen Patch

The transdermal estrogen patch was the first major development in HRT since conjugated estrogen. It was excellent news for women who needed estrogen desperately but couldn't take it orally because it can aggravate preexisting medical conditions such as gallbladder disease, liver impairment, renin-hypertension, or thrombophlebitis. An adhesive patch, it delivers estradiol at a controlled rate directly through the skin into the bloodstream. When estrogen does not pass through the digestive system and the liver, it does not cause the release of enzymes that could adversely affect those preexisting conditions.

Patches, rather than pills, are also commonly prescribed for smokers as well as women with high levels of triglycerides, although if the HDL level goes down after menopause, pills are best.

Research at nine major medical centers in the United States has shown that the transdermal system is just as safe and effective as oral estrogen. Approved by the FDA for the treatment of menopausal symptoms and prevention of osteoporosis, it also reverses the vaginal and urinary changes.

The patch is applied to clean dry skin on the abdomen, thigh, or buttocks and changed once or twice a week. Its only apparent side effect is occasional skin irritation from the adhesive. Many women have found, however, that this improves within a few weeks of use. If not, the patch won't lose its effectiveness if you pull it off and reapply it to a different spot when it becomes bothersome. The least sensitive area of the body is your buttocks, so if you have delicate skin, try it there.

And sometimes the patch comes off in the shower or the swimming pool. Just put it back on again. Or take it off while you shower or swim and reapply it when you come out. The water won't affect its efficacy. If you prefer, apply a new one, but stay on your same replacement schedule.

The first transdermal estrogen patch was approved by the FDA in the 1980s. Since then, several new varieties have become available. All of them deliver estradiol, the primary form of estrogen produced by the ovaries and the one that occurs naturally in plants. Affixed to the skin, the patch continuously releases tiny amounts of estradiol contained in a gel. This is absorbed through the skin, entering the capillaries and then traveling through the circulatory system to all parts of the body.

Many Patches Today

There are many varieties of estrogen patches now, and all of them will do the job, so whatever your gynecologist recommends is probably a good choice for you. On the other hand, you can always ask for a chance to try out other brands. Here's what is available at this writing.

Estraderm, the original estrogen patch, is changed twice a week and delivers estradiol in a choice of two dosages—0.05 mg (the equivalent of between 0.3 mg and 0.625 of conjugated estrogen); and 0.1 mg (the equivalent of between 0.9 and 1.25 mg of conjugated estrogen).

Vivelle is a matrix patch with the hormone embedded in the adhesive. Smaller, thinner, more flexible, and more transparent than Estraderm, it comes in four dosages: 0.0375 mg, 0.05 mg, 0.075 mg, and 0.1 mg. It is changed only once a week. Even newer is Vivelle-Dot, a tiny translucent patch the size of a small postage stamp. It is applied twice weekly and delivers the same four dosage strengths as the original Vivelle.

Climara, a once-a-week transdermal patch, offers estradiol in a very low 0.025 dose, as well as the more common amounts: 0.05 mg, 0.075 mg, and 0.1 mg. And Alora, changed two times a week, is marketed in two doses: 0.05 mg and 0.1 mg.

Combination Patch

Because women who have not had a hysterectomy and therefore still have a uterus must take progesterone along with estrogen, it is only logical that patches combining the two hormones are now on the market. Women who have been taking their estrogen by patch and their progesterone by pill can now get both together through their skin.

The CombiPatch, the first to be developed and approved by the FDA, delivers 0.05 mg of estradiol combined with progesterone in two doses, 0.14 mg and 0.25 mg. Changed twice a week and used every day of the month, it eliminates periods in about 75 percent of women because it inhibits the buildup of the uterine lining.

Vaginal Estrogen Cream

This is estrogen in cream form that is inserted into the vagina with a measured applicator. Although the hormone can be absorbed directly into the bloodstream and has some effect on other parts of the body, its main influence is on the tissues of the vagina and urethra where it reverses the atrophic changes caused by a deficiency of your own homemade estrogen.

So, in general, you should use this kind of estrogen replacement only for vaginal and urinary complaints. It should not be considered an equivalent to estrogen taken by pill or patch because it cannot be counted on to prevent osteoporosis or relieve severe menopausal symptoms. Besides, with this method of delivery, it is almost impossible to know how much of the hormone may be absorbed into the general circulation.

At first, the absorption is very rapid, sending peak amounts of hormones directly into the bloodstream. It then slows down after the vaginal epithelium has become recornified and thickened to a younger and healthier state.

Remember that you are on HRT when you use vaginal cream and you may also need to take progesterone as well, at least temporarily, if you have a uterus. So be sure to see your physician if you have any unplanned bleeding. Even if you don't have bleeding, it is essential to have regular endometrial biopsies, progesterone challenge tests, or ultrasound examinations to make sure you have not built up excessive lining because of the estrogen.

A major benefit of vaginal estrogen is that it does not aggravate such medical conditions as liver dysfunction, hypertension, gallbladder disease, and thrombophlebitis. Like transdermal estrogen, it is not absorbed through the digestive system and so it is not altered by the action of the liver.

The absorption of estrogen from vaginal cream varies widely, so you and your doctor will have to work out a schedule and a dose that's right for you. In most cases, 1 gram two or three times a week is sufficient, although you will probably start off with a higher dose and then taper off after your tissues have returned to normal.

For more about vaginal estrogen cream's effect on your vagina, urethra, and your sex life, see Chapters 8 and 9.

Vaginal Ring

An alternate route to delivering estrogen to the vagina is with a flexible time-release estrogen ring called Estring which is inserted much like a diaphragm. Like the patches, it releases minute amounts of estradiol continuously. It has the same effect as the creams, but can be left in place for three months.

Estring is very useful for women who don't wish to take the usual estrogen replacement but want to restore their vaginas to good working condition. Its estrogen is not absorbed into the bloodstream and circulated to the rest of the body; instead it goes only to the vagina. Therefore, it is an excellent way to help women who cannot use estrogen because of previous breast cancer. Just to make certain it is not entering the general circulation, however, it is a good idea in this case for your gynecologist to measure your blood for estrogen after a couple of months on the ring.

Another category of women who often find the vaginal ring a godsend are those who take Fosamax and Raloxifene for osteoporosis. Neither of these bone-building drugs help dry vaginas and, in fact, may make them worse.

DETERMINING THE RIGHT ESTROGEN DOSE

Always take the lowest amount of any drug, including estrogen, that will do the job assigned to it. In the case of estrogen, the smallest dose that will accomplish its purposes is the most you should use because you do not want to overstimulate the uterine lining.

Conjugated estrogen is available in five dosages, starting with 0.3 mg. If you can get by on 0.3 mg, fine, but few women can. Besides, if you are taking estrogen to protect your bones against osteoporosis, you probably require a minimum of 0.625 mg of conjugated estrogen or its equivalent to prevent bone loss, enough in most cases too for effectively relieving hot flashes and the other assorted symptoms.

We still recommend 0.625 mg for most women, although a study by researchers at Creighton University in Omaha suggests that a daily dose of only 0.3 mg may be enough to increase bone mineral density in women over 65 when adequate vitamin D and calcium are also taken. This is good news for women who suffer from unpleasant side effects when they take higher doses of estrogen.

If your hot flashes aren't banished by 0.625 mg, however, you can take 0.9 mg or even 1.25 mg (or its equivalent) and still remain in the low-dose range. A study has shown that low-dose Estrace (0.5 mg) can prevent osteoporosis, but may not be enough to relieve severe menopausal symptoms.

Sometimes you may need estrogen by pill or patch *plus* an occasional application of vaginal cream to keep your vaginal tissues in good condition.

Why Doses Differ

Every woman has her own individual requirements for estrogen that depend, among other things, on her weight, age, and the efficiency of her estrogen receptors that make her more or less sensitive to the effects of the hormone.

The usual dose is 0.625 mg of conjugated estrogen (or its equivalent), the minimum usually required to prevent bone loss and the amount usually necessary to alleviate the other atrophic changes caused by menopause. Most women do fine on that amount and that's what your gynecologist will probably start you off with. But some women need as little as 0.3 mg or the equivalent to banish hot flashes, while others require more. Women who have menopause at a young age, especially if it was an abrupt surgical menopause, often require more estrogen, perhaps 0.9 mg or even 1.25 mg, at least at the beginning. So do those with serious vaginal atrophy who need the higher dose until their tissues have been restored to a healthy condition.

Once or Twice a Day?

Oral estrogen is almost always taken just once a day. Occasionally, though, if your symptoms are extremely uncomfortable, you may find it more effective to divide the dose, taking half in the morning and the other half at night. This gives you an estrogen boost twice a day and promotes a more constant blood level of the hormone through the entire 24 hours. Transdermal patches, worn all day every day, also maintain a relatively constant hormone level.

DETERMINING THE RIGHT PROGESTERONE DOSE

Progesterone, the other important female hormone that should be taken in addition to estrogen by women who have not had hysterectomies, must be taken for a minimum of 10 days a month if it's going to protect your uterus. It is usually prescribed in doses of 5 mg for 12 to 14 days, or 10 mg for 10 to 12 days a month. Or, as we have described, it can be taken in low doses (usually 2.5 mg) every day of the month if this works better for you.

Not everyone gets along well on the standard doses and schedules, however, and the treatment must be individualized specifically for you, an excellent reason for seeing your gynecologist every six months or whenever your monthly bleeding doesn't follow its usual pattern. If you bleed heavily after your cyclical progesterone each month, or if you develop hyperplasia, then you require more progesterone than usual because you are superresponsive to estrogen. Or you may do better if your dose is stretched over more days per month, perhaps as many as 13, 14, or 15.

Your other option is to switch to the continuous progesterone pattern, taking progesterone in small doses every day of the month. If this doesn't work, you must go back to a cyclical pattern.

Although medroxyprogesterone (Provera) is the most common progesterone prescribed today, there are other kinds that your gynecologist may prefer. These include generic medroxyprogesterone, yam- or soybean-derived micronized progesterone, 19 nor-steroids such as Aygestin, and Crinone, a vaginal gel.

Progesterone After a Hysterectomy?

There's no reason to take progesterone if you have had a hysterectomy. The purpose of including it in HRT is to protect the uterus and you no longer have one.

FORGETTING YOUR PILLS

Forgetting to take your HRT pills for a couple of days isn't the same as forgetting to take birth control pills. If you skip birth control pills for a day, and certainly if you skip two days, you can assume you are not covered for that entire month and you'd better use other protection against pregnancy.

But don't worry if you miss a day or two of hormone replacement. It won't disturb the cycle and you will undoubtedly get the message to start again from a few unexpected hot flashes or some breakthrough bleeding. The same is true for the transdermal patch. Forgetting to change it for a couple of extra days won't do any harm, although it's wise not to make a habit of it.

If you miss more than a couple of days, however, and you experience no vasomotor symptoms, it may mean you don't need HRT to relieve symptoms anymore. They are gone. So, if your plan is to use the hormones only as long as you have symptoms, this is the time to see your physician to talk about quitting.

HRT ONLY NOW AND THEN?

Is it acceptable to take hormones only occasionally, perhaps once or twice a week? Or only when symptoms become troublesome? The answer is, it is never a good idea to take hormones (except for vaginal cream) only occasionally or on an irregular schedule if you have not had a hysterectomy and therefore still have your uterus. That's because this practice may cause an incomplete endometrial buildup and the lining will not be cleared out regularly by progesterone. The result may be bleeding or other problems and you are looking for trouble. Take your low dose every day (or twice a week for the patch) plus your progesterone as scheduled. Or stop taking it altogether. If you can get along with so little hormone, you can probably manage without any at all.

On the other hand, it isn't so important to maintain a regular schedule of estrogen if you have had a hysterectomy and therefore have no uterine lining to affect.

DOUBLE DOSE BY MISTAKE?

If you don't have a scheduled time of day to take your estrogen pill, you may occasionally take two in one day by mistake, maybe one after breakfast and another at night because you forgot about the first. It won't hurt you if you don't make a habit of it and end up overdosing yourself.

The best time to take your pill is just before bed. If you always take it when you brush your teeth at night, you will remember, and you will know you haven't taken one earlier that day. The same applies to your progesterone tablets.

As for the transdermal patch, it's doubtful you will apply a second one. However, you might forget to change it once or twice a week. So make yourself a schedule—say, every Monday, or every Monday and Thursday nights just before bed—and make sure you apply a new patch then. Post the schedule over your bathroom sink to remind you. Again, all is not lost if you forget. You'll remember when you start getting symptoms again.

SWITCHING FROM THE PILL

Now that the doses of some birth control pills are so low (even though they contain more estrogen than the usual HRT), they may safely be used by women up to the age of 50 and are especially helpful during perimenopause. But taking the pill after that age or after menopause is not recommended, as we have explained.

Oral contraceptives won't prevent menopause but they will cause you to continue having periods because of the hormones they contain. So if you continue taking them, you won't know if you have had menopause, until eventually, probably around the age of 60, the endo-metrium will become completely inactive and the peri-ods will stop.

If you have had menopause when you quit, although the event has been disguised by the effects of the pill, you will probably experience very severe symptoms, much like you would after a surgical menopause, because of the abrupt withdrawal of estrogen from your bloodstream. If this happens, go to your gynecologist and get help.

IS IT EVER TOO LATE FOR HRT?

It is never too late for at least some of its benefits. At what-ever age you start using it, estrogen will stop further bone loss, although it can't restore the bone you have already lost. It will provide some protection against cardiovascular disease by raising your HDL level and preserving the integrity of your arteries. It will rejuvenate your vaginal and urinary tissues, reconditioning your sex life and rais-ing your resistance to vaginal and urinary infections.

If you wait very many years before seeking estrogen's help, however, you may require a low dose of systemic estrogen at first while your body adjusts to the blood flow, and the beneficial results may take longer to occur.

Eventually the hormones will work, though perhaps not as well as they would have if you had taken them earlier. Sometimes long years of estrogen deficiency can cause such extensive degeneration of the tissues that they can never be completely restored. But in most cases you'd be amazed at what HRT can do.

REMEMBER YOUR CHECKUPS

When you are on HRT, you should have a checkup every six months. In fact, such a schedule is strongly advised whether or not you are on HRT. At each visit, the routine examination should include complete pelvic and breast examinations plus a Pap smear. Once a year, the doctor should also do blood tests.

If there is an indication of hyperplasia or other uterine problem, an aspiration biopsy is essential for examination of the endometrial cells. A Pap smear is *not* a reliable test of the endometrium because it retrieves only a sampling of cells from the vagina and cervix and none from the body of the uterus.

If you are taking long-term oral estrogen, the doctor should also be on the alert for possible aggravation of previous conditions such as renin-hypertension, liver dysfunction, gallbladder disease, or thrombophlebitis. These conditions are not affected by the patch.

HRT'S POSSIBLE SIDE EFFECTS

Hormone replacement therapy sometimes has its side effects. They are usually minor and transient or can be eliminated by switching to another dosage, form of hormone, schedule, or delivery system. But occasionally they are serious or uncomfortable enough to warrant abandoning the therapy. Most are completely reversible when the treatment is stopped.

Fluid Retention

This is the most common side effect and occurs in about half the women on HRT. Most of the time it only lasts a few weeks before vanishing. If it doesn't go away, you can probably get relief by cutting down on salt or taking an occasional mild diuretic. Try taking 100 to 500 mg a day of vitamin B_6, a natural diuretic. If that doesn't help enough, ask your doctor about aldactone (Spironolactone), a diuretic available by prescription. It is very mild and may be taken every day if necessary. Fluid retention isn't a serious complication, but about two in every 100 women consider it reason enough to quit the hormones.

Breast Tenderness

You may find your breasts become full and tender soon after you start taking estrogen, just as they did before your menstrual periods. This is almost always a temporary condition and nothing to worry about. The discomfort results from fluid retention and stimulated mammary glands, and it usually fades away or at least becomes tolerable within a few weeks. But sometimes it doesn't and can be a reason to stop HRT or to try the lowest possible dose.

For some women, taking progesterone over more days or continuously in low doses every day will take care of the problem. For others, switching to a different type of progesterone (19 nor-steroids, for example) eliminates the tenderness. As for estrogen, you might do best taking your estrogen cyclically, three weeks on, one week off, rather than continuously, to give yourself a respite once a month. Another option is to take estrogen in combination with a tiny dose of testosterone, a male hormone that women also produce in their ovaries and adrenals. This may relieve painfully tender breasts and, as an added bonus, improve your libido. Ask your gynecologist about trying this form of estrogen replacement marketed as Estratest. See Chapter 8 for more about it.

By the way, although physicians once warned women away from HRT if they had fibrocystic breast disease, we now know that this is not a precancerous condition and, besides, taking estrogen will not increase your chances of developing breast cancer. If the hormones cause additional discomfort, which is not likely because the dose is so small, discuss the options above with your doctor.

Weight Gain

About a quarter of the women who take estrogen report a gain of a few pounds when they first start HRT. This is probably the result of fluid retention and estrogen's tendency to encourage fat tissue, just as male hormones encourage muscle tissue.

But don't pin the blame for a big weight gain on your hormones. We all have a natural tendency to put on pounds as we get older because our metabolism slows down. At the same time, we also lose muscle mass and gain fat tissue.

Nausea

Many women suffer from mild nausea when they start taking oral estrogen, but this is almost always a transient side effect that wears off in a few weeks. Try taking your estrogen just before bed so you'll sleep through it. If the nausea doesn't improve, switch to the transdermal estrogen patch that delivers estrogen through the skin instead of the digestive system.

Vaginal Discharge

For some women, taking hormones can cause a supersupply of vaginal lubrication. This has no medical consequence but it certainly can be a nuisance. Douching with a mild solution of water and vinegar may help.

Headaches

Once in a while, women complain that hormone supplements give them headaches, especially if they already have a tendency to get migraines. The explanation may be that estrogen can cause blood vessels to dilate or spasm or induce the brain to retain fluid. Sometimes the headaches come from a low estrogen level on the week you take no estrogen when you use it cyclically.

You may have to engage in some trial and error to find a solution to this problem. Some women find they can prevent migraines by switching to the estrogen patch instead of taking pills, or, if the headaches are precipitated by a low estrogen blood level, by taking their pills every day of the month instead of cyclically. Sometimes, too, taking a lower dose or taking estrogen combined with a tiny dose of testosterone will eliminate the headache. Or try switching the type of estrogen you take from conjugated estrogen to pure estradiol or pure estrone.

If your headaches seem to be caused by progesterone, try the continuous method, taking very low doses every day of the month.

Allergic Reactions

It is possible to be allergic to almost anything, and occasionally a woman is allergic to estrogen supplements. They can cause rashes, swollen tongue, itching, all the typical allergic responses. Sometimes a different brand or method of estrogen replacement will solve the problem, but sometimes the only answer is to quit.

Skin Reactions

Some women find that the transdermal estrogen patch causes skin irritation, redness, and itching, although this is much less common today than it once was. If this happens to you, try taking the patch off and reapplying it in a different place. Make sure you apply it to dry skin after air-drying the patch for a few seconds when you remove it from its packaging. Try, too, wearing it on your buttocks where the skin is less sensitive than your abdomen.

Drug Sensitivity

In rare instances, oral estrogen heightens the sensitivity to certain other drugs that are also cleared by the liver. Simply switch to the transdermal patch.

HRT FOREVER?

You can safely take hormone therapy for a lifetime if you remember the important guidelines: low doses, progesterone if you haven't had a hysterectomy, a checkup every six months or whenever you have unscheduled bleeding, mammograms once a year. Many women need estrogen for the rest of their lives, especially if they are at high risk for osteoporosis or heart disease. Others need it to preserve their sex lives and prevent recurring vaginal and urinary infections.

When you take long-term hormone therapy, there is no need to stop the hormones for "a rest" no matter how many years go by, unless you develop side effects or hyperplasia.

Time to Quit?

If you are taking HRT only long enough to get through your menopausal symptoms comfortably, you probably won't need it for more than about two years. But you'll never know whether it's time to stop until you try it. Taper off the supplements gradually, as explained below, and see if the symptoms return. If they do, you may want to continue the estrogen (and progesterone, of course) for a while longer until you can stop without major discomfort.

Do You Lose the Benefits?

When you stop taking HRT, you lose the benefits it provides, although in the meantime you have gained a few years of protection against bone loss and heart disease.

Quitting HRT

Never quit hormones abruptly or you may find yourself overwhelmed with severe symptoms because of the rebound response from the hypothalamus. This can happen no matter how long you have been on HRT or whether you were still having symptoms before you began it. The sudden loss of estrogen deprives the estrogen receptors in the hypothalamus and causes it to produce an epinephrinelike substance that derails your temperature-regulating mechanism and results in hot flashes.

Always quit HRT very gradually. Cut back to every other day and hold it there for a month. Then take the pills only twice a week for a month, then once a week for a few more weeks before stopping altogether.

Don't taper off on progesterone, however. Continue to take your usual amount throughout the withdrawal before quitting it too.

If you no longer need estrogen for symptoms, you probably won't get them now. But if you do, you'll know it soon enough and you can always start taking the hormones again if you want to.

Don't Doctor Yourself

Don't try to be your own doctor when you take hormone replacement therapy—or any other drugs, for that matter. You need a knowledgeable and competent physician to write prescriptions, alter your treatment if necessary, and, most important, check out your reproductive health twice a year.

Remember this is your one and only body. If you want it to last a lifetime in good operating condition, you must take the best possible care of it.

8

SUPER SEX FOREVER

• •

Taking estrogen doesn't mean you are guaranteed a great sex life or that all your fantasies will come true. But without it, you may soon have no sex life at all. Estrogen is responsible for maintaining the size, shape, and flexibility of your vagina, as well as the thickness and lubrication of its lining. When you don't produce much of it anymore, physical changes take place that can make sex become uncomfortable, downright painful, or even totally impossible.

Astonishingly few women know these facts of life about sex after estrogen. When their difficulties begin, they are often too embarrassed to talk about them even to their doctors. Most women wait until sex has become miserable before seeking help, or even finding out that help is out there, and a good percentage simply assume their sex lives are over. But spread the word. This is one problem that is easily and rapidly resolved with HRT and has become the main reason why women make the decision to take it.

Estrogen restores vaginal tissues to a more youthful state, thicker, moister, more flexible. Even for women who are already in deep sexual difficulty, the therapy usually reverses the damage in only a few weeks.

That does not mean every women must take hormone replacement therapy after menopause. Some women don't need it, at least for several years. For one thing, there really is truth in the warning, "Use it or lose it." An active sex life helps the sex organs remain in good working condition. Besides, you may be among those few fortunate women who continue to manufacture enough estrogen throughout their lives to keep these tissues functioning for many years.

However, virtually every woman will have to give up sexual intercourse eventually unless she starts taking estrogen.

The ability to have and enjoy sex lasts for a lifetime. It's never gone, although many women cease to use it. So, assuming you have a compatible partner or the prospect of one, there is no reason not to help yourself enjoy sex again. Taking HRT is not going to give you cancer and it may pave the way to a super sex life.

HOW LONG WILL IT TAKE?

Although some women have uncomfortable intercourse only four to six months after menopause (especially after a surgical menopause), it usually takes 3 to 10 years from the time you lose your primary estrogen source before the typical vaginal problems become acute.

That's why you are lucky if you have a late menopause—these changes will happen much later in your life. A woman who has menopause at 55, for example, will probably not experience serious difficulties until she is about 60 or 65. But if your menopause takes place at 35, you will be in sexual trouble at a much earlier age, perhaps at 38 or 45, unless you take estrogen.

HORMONES AND YOUR LIBIDO

Passing the milestone of menopause doesn't seem to affect sexual desire or orgasmic ability one way or the other for most women. Some women, however, find they are *more* interested now that they're not concerned about getting pregnant and have fewer inhibitions and consuming responsibilities. In addition, libido may even increase as the male hormones every woman makes become more influential without the counterbalance of estrogen. Many women experience a real sexual reawakening at this time of their lives and it is not unusual for someone who never before experienced orgasms to begin now.

Other women find their interest in sex wanes with menopause. One good reason is that the physical changes can certainly take their toll on the joy of sex. But interest diminishes very often, too, because women think they *should* be less active and that sex is appropriate only for the young. Some of them, of course, don't have a partner who turns them on. Others have never cared much for sex anyway and use menopause as a convenient excuse to forget it.

The story may be different if your testosterone level is very low, especially when it drops because of having had your ovaries removed or irrevocably damaged. All women produce androgens, male hormones, mainly in their ovaries but with an additional small amount made by the adrenal glands. One of these hormones, testosterone, fuels the sex drive in both men and women. When its level plummets, so does libido.

Even with a natural menopause, the production of this hormone decreases by nearly 50 percent. But if your ovaries have been removed or severely damaged, causing a precipitous and almost total drop in testosterone, you may suffer a much more dramatic loss of interest in sex.

A shortage of androgens, easily detected by a simple blood test, can not only decrease libido and orgasmic ability, but can also induce depression and lethargy. If your problems prove to result from an androgen deficiency, there's an easy answer. Tiny doses of testosterone can help rekindle your sexual desire, accomplishing its goal within only a few days. It is usually taken orally, alone or in combination with estrogen, intermittently for several days at a time. An added benefit is that the male hormone relieves the breast tenderness experienced by some women on estrogen. Don't worry—you won't grow a mustache. You'll find more information about testosterone later in this chapter.

By the way, although there is still some controversy about this, some cancer specialists see no reason to prohibit testosterone treatment for women with breast cancer if they have lost libido because of an androgen deficiency. Substitutes for testosterone, although not as effective, include the drugs Wellbutrin and Eldeporil. Megace, a form of progesterone, also may help increase libido.

THE UNIVERSAL PHYSICAL CHANGES

All women who are a few years past menopause experience vaginal changes, if they don't take HRT. Unlike the early symptoms such as hot flashes that eventually disappear with or without help, these changes gradually progress with time. Blood flow to the genitals decreases. It takes longer to become sexually aroused and longer as well to produce lubrication in preparation for intercourse. Sensory perception diminishes and the external genitalia lose their subcutaneous layer of fat. The vagina becomes dryer, narrower, less pliable and expandable, maybe even a little shorter. In some cases, the entrance narrows so much that it won't allow intercourse at all. The vaginal lining loses its tough protective layer of cornified cells and becomes thinner, smoother, less elastic, less acidic, more easily irritated and susceptible to infections. It also loses its thick cushiony rugal folds that allowed for elasticity and expansion.

If you don't want these changes to affect your sexual activities, you are going to have to deal with them one way or another. Don't be afraid to discuss your problems with your gynecologist because *you need help*. Many women are still reluctant to talk about such subjects and, unfortunately, many doctors are reluctant to bring them up. But force yourself to be open and frank so you can get on with your sex life.

Loss of Lubrication

A vagina that is dry and unlubricated can definitely be a deterrent to sexual enjoyment. This is the first sign of vaginal change and it usually becomes noticeable very soon after, and sometimes before, menopause. When estrogen no longer stimulates the production of cervical and vaginal mucus, the vagina loses much of the lubrication needed for comfortable intercourse. Women who lose estrogen very slowly and continue to make some for many years don't find dryness much of a problem in the early years, but most women do.

When lack of lubrication remains your only problem, it can easily be overcome in most cases with lubricants and moisturizers made for this purpose. See below for details.

By the way, antihistamines and decongestants that are designed to dry nasal membranes also tend to dry vaginal membranes. So do other drugs, including cardiovascular medications, antidepressants, atropine drugs, and diuretics.

The Easily Irritated Vagina

The second vaginal problem caused by an estrogen deficit is the thinning of the vaginal lining. Without estrogen stimulation, the lining gradually becomes thinner and less elastic, so it is easily irritated or broken and may even bleed.

An easily irritated and inflamed lining can obviously lead to uncomfortable intercourse and a minimal interest in sex. In fact, when the lining becomes so thin that it is virtually nonexistent, sexual intercourse becomes so painful that it is impossible. At that point, it is essential to start estrogen therapy unless you are willing to give up intercourse forever.

In addition to providing a happy home for infectious organisms, the thin, dry lining sometimes develops a chronic noninfectious inflammation called atrophic vaginitis. Spotting from this kind of inflammation necessitates biopsies and D&Cs (dilation and curettage) for thousands of women a year because *any* bleeding requires investigation.

The thinning occurs because an important function of estrogen is to stimulate the creation of a tough outer layer of cornified cells that protect the more delicate underlying tissues against injury and infection. This thickened epithelium develops at puberty and vanishes with menopause, the reason why little girls and old women are especially susceptible to vaginal infection. See the next chapter for more about infections and what to do about them.

A sidelight: The same kind of layer of cornified epithelium covering the entire vagina is also found in the mouth and nose. This tissue, too, tends to thin and dry when your estrogen goes.

Urinary inflammation and infections are other problems that occur for the very same reason. The protective outer layer of the urethral lining also thins out with the loss of estrogen. This means the urethra, located adjacent to the vagina, can be easily irritated and injured especially during sexual activity, and so it becomes more susceptible to infectious organisms. The bladder, also estrogen-dependent, loses much of its elasticity as well. See the next chapter for more about the urinary tract.

The Changing Shape of the Vagina

Without estrogen, the vagina reverts to its prepubertal state in another way. It becomes shorter and narrower and its walls become less elastic. Added to the loss of lubrication and the thinning of the lining, these changes can definitely affect your attitude toward making love.

HOW AN ACTIVE SEX LIFE HELPS

Frequent sexual intercourse keeps the vagina more elastic, flexible, and lubricated. According to Masters and Johnson, intercourse at least once or twice a week over a period of years will help keep a woman of any age more interested and able. The stimulation encourages the production of mucus secretions, helps to maintain muscle tone and preserve the shape and size of the vagina.

That's why sexually active women often have a few years' grace, delaying the inevitable changes until a little later in their lives. But eventually they too will have the same dysfunctions other women have, unless they use estrogen.

Sexual Variations

The standard kind of sexual activity—intercourse—is not the only way to help keep yourself in good working order, although it is the best. Any method of achieving orgasm, including masturbation, can retard the atrophic changes.

If this embarrasses you, remember that attitudes have changed and gynecologists today are seeing many more women than ever for sexual problems. In former days, women who had difficulties because of an estrogen deficit simply accepted their supposedly inevitable fate and gave up sex or the hope of it. Today they look for help. If you need it, do the same.

DIABETES AND SEX

Diabetic women tend to have more sexual difficulties after menopause than women with normal blood sugar levels. They often experience a marked reduction in lubrication and sexual desire, and when their glucose levels are high, their vaginal secretions provide the perfect environment for yeast infections.

HOW TO HELP YOURSELF

Let's save the discussion of hormone replacement therapy for last and talk first about other ways to fend off sexual suicide.

Lubricants

In the early years after menopause when your only difficulty may be vaginal dryness, you can probably do very well with a personal lubricant such as Surgilube, K-Y Jelly, Astroglide, Lubrin, Maxilube, Transilube, or Ortho Personal Lubricant, to prevent the uncomfortable friction of intercourse. If you need more help, you may want to use vaginal suppositories, such as Lubrin Vaginal Lubricating Inserts or Lubafax, in addition to the lubricants. They are inserted into the vagina where they quickly dissolve.

Never use a lubricant that is not designed for vaginal lubrication, because it can compound your problems.

Most cosmetic creams, for example, contain perfume and alcohol that can irritate tender tissues. Don't use petroleum jelly or baby oil because they may cake and dry, causing irritation or damage, provide a habitat for bacteria, and block the release of your own secretions as well. Besides, they can also destroy latex condoms and damage diaphragms. The lubricant you use must be water-soluble and oil-free.

The only exception is vitamin E oil, which doesn't dry or cake and may possibly have a beneficial effect on the vaginal lining. Stay away from almond oil, coconut oil, or other flavored oils. Their high sugar content encourages fungal infections.

Moisturizers

Even more effective than lubricants are nonhormonal moisturizing gels such as Replens and Gyne-Moistrin that are sold over the counter. They hydrate the cells of the vaginal lining and allow them to build up a continually moist protective layer, significantly increasing moisture, acidity, and elasticity in most cases after a few months. The gels work well for women who can't take, or don't choose to take, HRT. They are nowhere near as effective as estrogen because they don't restore the protective cornified layer of the vaginal lining. But they can help by temporarily plumping up the cells of the lining with moisture, making it less dry and irritable. Each application lasts up to three days. The moisturizer is inserted into the vagina with a disposable applicator about three times a week, preferably in the morning.

The newest moisturizer around is Vagisil Intimate Moisturizer. A natural nonhormonal product, it can be used for the vulva, the external portion of the vagina, which sometimes becomes very dry and irritable, and also for the vagina when used internally. It is sold over the counter.

A big advantage of the moisturizers is that they have a very low pH, meaning they are acidic and therefore help to maintain a healthy vaginal environment where unfriendly bacteria are not likely to flourish.

Don't use them as lubricants. They don't do a good lubricating job and, besides, their acidity may make them irritating to your partner's tissues.

Vitamin Therapy

Whether vitamin supplements will affect sexual desire or performance is debatable, but vitamin E has been credited with beneficial effects and so have the B vitamins. Of course, it is essential too to keep your body in good shape with a healthy diet, sufficient exercise, and plenty of rest.

HRT AND YOUR SEX LIFE

If you are suffering from uncomfortable vaginal changes, you are strongly urged to start hormone replacement therapy, the ultimate answer, if there is no medical reason you can't. It has saved untold numbers of marriages and relationships and made others possible.

Only a minimal amount of estrogen is required in most cases to prevent or remedy every one of the changes we have described and make sex comfortable again, and you will start seeing results in only a couple of weeks. There is nothing else yet discovered that will do the same job of rejuvenating these tissues.

The lining will start thickening; lubrication will increase; the tenderness, itchiness, and soreness will be alleviated. By five or six weeks, you will probably be as good as new, although if you have really let yourself go before seeking treatment, it may take a few months to see real improvement.

The estrogen dose must be individualized because some women require more estrogen than others to produce the same results. Always stay with a low dose, however, and do not fail to take progesterone too if you have a uterus. Every woman's vagina can be restored to mint condition with enough estrogen, but the high doses some women need to accomplish perfect results are too high for safety. If this is the case with you, you may have to accept a compromise. But don't worry—there will always be remarkable improvement and you will be in much better shape than you were before. The criteria for successful treatment with HRT are comfortable sex and no more than one or two vaginal or urinary infections a year.

Are You Ever Beyond Repair?

No matter how long your vagina has been out of commission because of lack of estrogen, it will almost invariably regenerate with therapy. Even if you have been living without estrogen for decades, your tissues will probably be restored to a functional condition after only a few weeks or sometimes a few months of treatment.

When Your Partner Takes Viagra

It's a whole new world for many older women when their husbands or partners, formerly unable to manage intercourse, start taking Viagra. Some women have lost interest in sex or become accustomed to other ways of being sexually satisfied. Many have developed nonfunctioning vaginas and haven't bothered treating them. If this is happening to you, make haste to your gynecologist's office and get going on hormone replacement therapy. Until its effects kick in, you can get a quick fix with vaginal estrogen cream or an estrogen ring. Meanwhile, use a vaginal moisturizer and/or lubricant to ease the situation.

Viagra for Women?

The first preliminary study on the effects of Viagra on women with sexual dysfunction found that it had little, if any, effect. Even if it did work, by the way, it does not appear to do anything that estrogen can't do.

Viagra and Urinary Infections

An unexpected side effect of the anti-impotence drug Viagra is the likelihood of urinary tract infections in women shortly after sexual relations are resumed. The reason, of course, is that most women whose partners take this drug are postmenopausal and therefore—unless they take hormone replacement—suffer from estrogen-deficient vaginal and urethral linings, which make them susceptible to vaginal and urinary infections. See Chapter 9.

PILLS, PATCHES, CREAMS, AND RINGS

There are four major kinds of hormone replacement therapy, and each has its advantages and advocates. We will describe them here again and focus on their relationship with your vaginal tissues.

VAGINAL ESTROGEN CREAM

If your only postmenopausal problems are vaginal and/or urinary, you will probably do fine with vaginal estrogen cream as your replacement therapy. The topical estrogens are absorbed by the vaginal tissues, reversing the degenerative changes, recornifying and thickening the lining, encouraging lubrication, and relieving dryness. In only a few days, the cornified cells will start to make a reappearance.

How much cream and how often you use it depends on your own individual requirements. Some women need more than the usual dose because they don't absorb it as efficiently as other women. So it may take some trial and error to find out what's right for you.

Except in unusual cases, it's best to begin with a relatively high dose, perhaps 2 grams three times a week for two weeks, and then cut back to 1 gram twice a week. It is nonproductive to use too much because the vagina will absorb only as much estrogen as it needs. At first when your tissues are very dry and thin, they will absorb a much greater amount than they will later on after they have been restored to good condition.

You can maintain your own schedule with vaginal cream, starting and stopping it as necessary. Some women use it only temporarily until they have improved and then go back to lubricants alone. That's acceptable, although they will inevitably have to resume the treatment after a few months. The symptoms always return when the therapy is stopped and therefore this must be a lifetime commitment.

Although you may decide to use the estrogen cream just before intercourse because it gives some local lubrication, this is a waste of the medication. It's best to apply it when you are not anticipating sex to give it time to work and avoid having it absorbed by your partner. Besides, the lubricants made for this purpose do a much better job.

Remember, You're on Hormones

Don't think when you use vaginal cream that you are not on hormone therapy. This *is* a form of HRT. Some of the estrogen you apply locally is absorbed into your bloodstream just like estrogen taken any other way. Although there is high absorption in the first few days before it decreases to a minimal amount after the lining is regenerated, you *are* taking estrogen and, just like any other estrogen, it *can* affect the rest of your body including the lining of your uterus.

That means you must see your doctor regularly to be sure you are not developing hyperplasia, an overproliferation of the endometrium that, untreated, can lead to uterine cancer. If you have hyperplasia, you must take progesterone too, at least periodically.

Report to your doctor between regular visits if you have any bleeding or spotting while you are using estrogen cream, even a low dose, because this may be a warning signal that trouble is brewing.

Even if you don't bleed when you use the cream, you should be sure you are really safe from excess proliferation of the lining by having a progesterone challenge test after you have been using vaginal cream for a few months. This means you take one course of progesterone—your gynecologist may prescribe 5 mg for 12 days of the month, or perhaps 10 mg for 10 days—while you continue to use the cream. If you bleed, it shows the estrogen is building up the lining and you should take progesterone on a regular monthly schedule. If you don't bleed, great. But be sure to continue testing yourself every few months.

Is Estrogen Cream Safe for Everyone?

The vaginal cream is considered safe as a short-term therapy even for women for whom estrogen has been ruled out for medical reasons. It may be used briefly and temporarily to relieve the worst symptoms and infections that refuse to respond to anything else. The treatment can not only banish some decidedly miserable chronic infections, but it can also restore the ability to have sexual intercouse. When the vaginal walls become extremely thin and rigid—as they inevitably do when there is no circulating estrogen—the lubricants and moisturizers won't work. Once the estrogen has restored the tissues, however, the lubricants will be effective enough until the next round of treatment becomes necessary.

We have found that only 1 gram of vaginal cream once a week will help to make the vagina more functional in women for whom the usual HRT has been ruled out because of estrogen-dependent breast cancer. Because this is such a tiny dose, it is most unlikely to be absorbed into the bloodstream where it might accelerate the growth of any remaining cancer cells. Of course, your blood estrogen levels should be checked regularly while you are on this regime.

A second possible solution in the future for breast cancer patients who can't take HRT in its usual forms is the vaginal estrogen ring, now used in Europe and awaiting approval in the United States. Worn in the vagina, it releases a steady but minute amount of estrogen daily, just enough to restore the vaginal tissues but not enough to be absorbed into the bloodstream.

VAGINAL RING

As we explained in the last chapter, the vaginal ring called Estring is another way to restore your vagina to good health. It is inserted into the vagina, much like a diaphragm, where it delivers a small dose of estrogen transdermally through the mucous membranes and need be changed only every three months. If you want to take estrogen solely to restore your vagina to good condition and you don't want to be bothered inserting vaginal cream regularly, this is a good choice.

The ring is an option, too, for women who can't take other kinds of estrogen because of earlier breast cancer because the hormone is not absorbed into the bloodstream but goes only to the vagina. It is also a great choice for women who take Fosamax or Raloxifene for osteoporosis. Neither of these drugs help dry vaginas that cause painful intercourse.

ORAL AND TRANSDERMAL ESTROGEN

If, in addition to solving your sexual problems, you need estrogen to protect your bones from osteoporosis or your heart from coronary artery disease, then you must take it long term by pill or by patch, perhaps occasionally supplemented by vaginal cream. The estrogen in vaginal cream is not absorbed in sufficient amounts to help your bones or your heart—or your skin either, for that matter. It won't even do much for hot flashes and other symptoms if they are more than mild.

Besides, it is almost impossible to know just how much of the hormone you are absorbing into the bloodstream, perhaps affecting the endometrium, when you take it by cream. Taken by pill or by patch, the dosage can be controlled.

Sometimes, when vaginal problems are severe, the results are best if you start off by taking estrogen by pill or patch and, at the same time, using the vaginal cream as well for a few weeks. This rejuvenates the membranes and resolves the difficulties very quickly. Then, if vaginal changes were your *only* concern, you can stop taking the pill or using the patch and continue using the cream as needed.

BACK TO YOUR LIBIDO

It may be wise to explore the possibility of taking testosterone only after you've tried other approaches to restoring your interest in sex. Without a doubt, estrogen therapy is the most effective way to get back into good physical working order, whether you choose oral, transdermal, vaginal estrogen creams or rings, or any other kind of estrogen replacement. And lubricants and moisturizers will help. It is not easy to enjoy intercourse when it hurts.

But, if all else is in order, and yet you have lost much of your sex drive, adding androgens to estrogen therapy may be your answer. The findings of a study published in 1998 by Philip Sarrell, M.D., of the Yale School of Medicine, offer strong evidence that combined estrogen-androgen is superior to estrogen alone in improving sexual sensation and desire.

So, if tests show that your testosterone level is low (under 30 mg per 100 ml), consider testosterone replacement, available in ointment, pills, lozenges, and, soon to come, transdermal patches. Estratest tablets, for example, combine 2.5 mg of testosterone with 1.25 mg of estrogen; or 1.25 mg of testosterone with 0.625 mg of estrogen. In most cases, the half-strength dose is enough.

REMEMBER YOUR GOALS

What you are trying to accomplish now is comfortable sex with no pain during intercourse and no more than one or two vaginal or urinary infections a year, tops. If these goals elude you, you may have to increase your estrogen dose. Make an appointment with your doctor to discuss the possibility, but never take more than 1.25 mg of conjugated estrogen or the equivalent a day except under very exceptional circumstances and under the supervision of your gynecologist.

9

No More Infections

• •

After menopause, when you run out of your major source of estrogen, you may find you're getting one vaginal or urinary infection after another. We are going to give you some sensible suggestions for preventing and coping with them, but your only hope for a real change in your uncomfortable situation is estrogen therapy, which rejuvenates the tissues of both the vagina and urethra, making them more resistant to infections. In fact, for women who get constant serious urinary infections that endanger their bladders and kidneys, HRT is absolutely essential.

WHY VAGINITIS NOW?

When your body lacks plentiful estrogen, the vaginal lining becomes dryer, thinner, less lubricated, and less elastic, making it more easily irritated and inflamed. The vagina gets tighter, sometimes shorter, and loses the rugal folds that allow it to expand and contract during intercourse. All of these happenings make it vulnerable to irritation and infection.

Contributing to the problem is a change in the vagina's pII or acidity balance. In your reproductive years, the normal pH of the vagina is acidic, although there are slight variations throughout the menstrual cycle. Most harmful bacteria and fungi are discouraged by an acidic environment, while the friendly flora that defend you against infection tend to flourish in it. When your estrogen level is low, however, the vagina becomes much more alkaline, providing a climate more hospitable to harmful organisms and less suitable for the helpful varieties. That's why women after menopause often get infection after infection and find, just when they've finished with one bout, they're faced with another.

URINARY INFECTIONS TOO

Urinary inflammations and infections also tend to become common occurrences for several reasons, all due to your altered anatomy and new hormonal status. For starters, the outermost portion of the urethra, located just above the vaginal opening, becomes less flexible and elastic with the loss of estrogen. At the same time, its covering membrane gets thinner, dryer, more irritable, and more attractive to infectious organisms that normally live in the intestinal tract.

In addition, because of the thinning of the vaginal walls, the urethra and bladder, located very close to the vagina, have less protection. That makes them subject to trauma, especially if you are sexually active. Compounding the problem, the distance between the vagina and urethra becomes shorter, allowing infections to cross over more easily from one to the other. At the same time, the bladder capacity is reduced as this inflatable organ becomes less elastic and its supports begin to sag. So no wonder you tend to be plagued with that familiar burning sensation during urination and a bladder that continually demands to be emptied.

WHAT TO DO

Restoring your vagina and urethra with HRT can do wonders if you suffer from constant infections and irritations because it will return the tissues to a more functional state that is not so attractive to hostile bacteria and other malevolent organisms. Of course, you will still get an occasional invasion, just as you did when you were younger, but you won't be in the same everlasting discomfort. So don't let your prejudices or your fears prevent you from helping yourself if you need estrogen badly. This is a valid reason for seriously considering hormones.

Vaginal estrogen cream applied locally may be all that's required. The cream helps by thickening the tissues, relieving the dryness and inelasticity, and encouraging lubrication. It also creates a more acidic environment. Even women for whom estrogen has been medically contraindicated can usually use vaginal cream intermittently for short periods of time to give them some relief from recurrent vaginal and urinary infections.

Estrogen taken orally or by transdermal patch has an even more dramatic effect on both the vagina and urethra because more of the hormone is absorbed and circulated to all the tissues of the body.

In most cases, a minimal estrogen dose does a good job of banishing infections, although every woman is different and some require more than others. So if you find when you are on HRT that you tend to get more than one or two infections a year, you may need a slight increase in dosage. Or you may get good results from applying vaginal cream now and then, in addition to your pills or patches. Discuss these possibilities with your physician.

A second choice, less effective than HRT, is to use a vaginal moisturizer such as Replens or Gyne-Moistrin regularly. One of its major attributes is that it is acidic and discouraging to harmful bacteria.

Never ignore infections because, while they are sometimes self-limiting, they usually get worse and more tenacious when left untreated. Make sure your physician makes the appropriate tests to determine which infection you have before giving you a prescription for an antibiotic or other medication. Never use a drug left over from an earlier infection without instructions from the doctor because it may not be appropriate now and can cost you time.

Remember to ask if your sexual partner should be treated too, since many infections are passed back and forth between partners.

Sometimes it is impossible for your physician to identify the organism that is causing a minor infection, making it impossible to prescribe the appropriate medication. Try douching with a nonprescription iodine preparation (Betadine), which may keep the offending bacteria under control.

More Ways to Help Prevent Vaginal Infections

First, keep yourself in good physical condition. Your immunity to the bacteria and other malevolent organisms that are always lurking around waiting for their next chance is diminished when you are rundown, tired, or undernourished.

Keep yourself scrupulously clean using mild nonperfumed soap and water. Always wipe yourself from front to back after a bowel movement to prevent intestinal bacteria from migrating to the vagina or urethra.

Keeping clean does not mean douching or spraying. Many commercial douches and feminine hygiene sprays are irritating and drying. They may also destroy the friendly organisms that prevent pathogens from multiplying. If you feel compelled to douche, do it no more than once a week with plain warm water.

If, however, you tend to get multiple infections because of the new alkaline condition of your vagina, you can use mild vinegar douches to help make it more acidic. Twice a week is plenty. Use a prepared vinegar solution, or make one yourself by mixing 1 tablespoon of vinegar in a quart of warm water. Your doctor may also prescribe medicinal douches for specific infections.

An occasional douche with baking soda (1 tablespoon to 1 quart of water) will help soothe the itching of fungal infections before they are cleared up.

Caution: Never hang a douche bag higher than a foot or so above your hips and never try to force the solution higher than it wants to go. This can wash organisms from the vagina into the uterus.

More Do's and Don'ts

• If you are not on HRT, use a nonhormonal vaginal moisturizer regularly to restore some protective moisture, thickness, and acidity to the vaginal lining (see Chapter 8).

• Use a vaginal lubricant during sexual intercourse to reduce the friction and help the tissues to stretch. Always use a lubricant designed specifically for this purpose and *never* use petroleum jelly, cosmetic creams, oils, or other substances that could make your problems worse. Again, see Chapter 8 for details.

• Wear cotton underpants or pants with cotton crotches. Synthetic fibers have been blamed for recurrent vaginitis because they don't allow air circulation, moisture evaporation, or drainage.

• Don't wear pants to bed. Don't wear pantyhose, tight jeans, or synthetic workout gear too much of the time.

• For the same reason, if you are still having periods, use sanitary pads instead of tampons. That allows more air to reach the vagina and avoids irritating the dry lining.

• Don't share. Because you can pick up organisms from other people, avoid using someone else's panties, bathing suit, towels, washcloths. Beware of hot tubs, even your own, if you have a tendency to get vaginitis. The infectious organisms flourish in the hot water and may choose you as their next victim. The chlorine that protects you in a swimming pool evaporates because of the heat of the hot tub's water.

• Choose your bed partners carefully. Insist on a condom (and spermicide) with a man you don't know well, haven't known long, or don't totally trust to be monogamous.

• Take antibiotics and penicillin only when necessary and under a doctor's supervision. They can upset the pH balance of the vagina, making it even more alkaline and inviting to hostile organisms. They may also destroy the friendly bacteria such as lactobacilli and leave you a likely candidate for fungal infections. Tetracycline is a chief offender, even when used only on the skin.

• Use an antifungal medication such as Monistat or Gyne-Lotrimin, now available without prescription, as a preventive if you get a yeast infection every time you take antibiotics. Start taking it the day you start the antibiotics and continue until you are finished.

• Some detergents and soaps can cause irritation. If you are constantly having problems, try switching brands.

• Check out your sugar intake. High blood sugar encourages fungal infections, the reason diabetics tend to get them.

• Eat at least a few ounces of live-culture yogurt every day to increase your lactobacilli, the friendly bacteria that help fight off the harmful organisms. Some women also swear by applications of yogurt in the vagina.

• Increase your consumption of vitamin C, which seems to help some women fight vaginal inflammation.

More Ways to Help Prevent Urinary Infections

Urinary tract infections (UTIs) are not only bothersome or even painful, but they can travel up the urethra to the bladder or the kidneys and become serious business. So it is very important to treat them promptly when you feel that familiar burning sensation. Whether or not you take estrogen, you can help yourself ward off infections by following these sensible suggestions:

• Wash with soap and water at least once a day, using a mild nonperfumed, nonirritating soap.

• Concentrated urine provides an excellent breeding ground for pernicious organisms, so keep your urine diluted by drinking plenty of fluids, preferably water, which is cheap, available, and noncaloric. Drink even more if you already have an infection.

• Make a practice of urinating at least several times a day without waiting for an urgent call. In fact, urinate as often as possible. And be sure to empty your bladder completely. If you can't do it in one sitting, wait for 10 minutes after urinating and then urinate again.

• Empty your bladder before sexual intercourse so it is less likely to suffer trauma. Empty it immediately afterward to prevent bacteria from migrating into the urinary track. Use a water-soluble vaginal lubricant during intercourse (see Chapter 8).

• Drink cranberry or blueberry juice, both of which have been found to contain compounds that help prevent bacteria from sticking to the walls of the bladder and urethra. Drink 4 to 8 ounces spaced out through the day.

• Avoid vaginal sprays or douches (except for plain water or mild vinegar-and-water solutions) because they tend to be irritating and drying.

• Monitor what you eat and drink, consuming more fruits and vegetables to make the urine more acidic, and less high-fat foods, which produce a more alkaline urine. Limit your alcohol consumption because alcohol dehydrates your body and concentrates the urine. Try eliminating caffeine and spicy foods, which can act as irritants to the urethra.

• Remember that physical trauma to the urethra during strenuous sexual activity is a common cause of irritation and UTIs. And try to avoid sexual activities that may move bacteria from the anal area to the vagina (and therefore the urethra).

MORE TRIPS TO THE BATHROOM

If you are making more trips to the bathroom both day and night, here's the reason why. The estrogen-deficient bladder loses much of its elasticity and holds less urine, which means you feel the urge to urinate more frequently.

Leaky Bladders

Stress incontinence—involuntary urinating that can be triggered by a sneeze, a laugh, an orgasm, a hop, a jump, or sometimes hardly anything at all—is a very common female problem. In fact, it's been estimated that as many as 40 percent of women over 45 have it, at least occasionally. In most cases, it begins before menopause and then gradually gets worse.

A leaky bladder is not a disease but a symptom of an underlying condition that can almost always be corrected or at least mitigated. The most common cause, especially among women who have had vaginal deliveries that have permanently weakened the pelvic muscles and supports, is a sagging bladder and urethra. Add to that the effects of age and menopause. With the loss of estrogen, the bladder loses muscle tone and elasticity, making it less able to hold as much urine as it once did.

Incontinence may also be caused by such things as urinary infections, inflammation, large fibroids, certain medications such as antihypertensives and antidepressants, obesity, previous pelvic surgery, even severe constipation.

What to do about a leaky bladder? Treat the underlying condition and your problem may be solved, but don't wait, as most women do, until life has become difficult. Tell your doctor about it and have a thorough examination to determine the cause and the treatment. Your primary physician or gynecologist may have the expertise to perform some or all of the appropriate tests and then treat you, but in most cases you will probably be referred to a specialist.

Try HRT First

Estrogen replacement is the first line of treatment to consider when incontinence occurs after menopause because it can restore the bladder and urethra to a state that's a lot closer to its former self and more able to defend itself against infections and other assaults. If you can't or don't want to take estrogen systemically, then at least try vaginal estrogen cream, the effects of which are almost totally limited to this specific part of your body.

Other measures prescribed by your physician may include muscle-strengthening exercises, elimination of certain drugs, bladder training, clearing up infections, medications, injections, and surgery.

Tighten Up with Exercise

Try to strengthen the sphincter of the bladder and the muscles of the pelvic floor that surround the urethra and vagina. Exercise can alleviate mild cases of stress incontinence and, at the same time, tone up the vagina.

Every time you think of it, as many times a day as possible, tighten the muscles as if you were trying very hard to hold back your urine. Tighten, hold for 10 seconds, relax, at least 20 times per session.

Or here's another way to do it. Every time you urinate, start the flow, then stop before you're finished. Holding back, count slowly to 10, then let go. Repeat several times.

Vaginal cones provide an alternative method of exercising the sphincter and the pelvic floor. The cones, used in gradually increasing weights, are inserted into the vagina. Then, in your efforts to hold them in, you train yourself to contract and strengthen the muscles.

Urge Incontinence

This kind of incontinence is caused by a bladder that tends to contract without your permission at inopportune moments and is not likely to be affected by hormone therapy. Caused by uncontrolled contractions of the bladder's detrusor muscle as it fills with urine, its symptoms often include a sudden overwhelming urge to urinate, urination eight or more times in 24 hours, and sudden unexpected release of urine.

The usual treatment is medication to relax the contractions, combined with bladder training, which teaches you to urinate at scheduled times only. Detrol, the first drug specifically designed to treat overactive bladder, was approved by the FDA in 1999. Causing fewer side effects such as dryness and palpitations than earlier medications for this problem, it works by inhibiting bladder sensitivity so you don't respond constantly to the small contractions that make you feel you have a full bladder. Take it twice a day or, if your problem occurs only at night, take it just once at bedtime.

Other Ways to Help Yourself

Meanwhile, consume a lot of fluids because highly concentrated urine is irritating to the bladder and likely to encourage infections. Try to keep your bladder as empty as possible by urinating at every possible opportunity. Lose weight if you are obese. Stop smoking. Avoid colored or perfumed toilet paper, perfumed soaps, detergent bath additives. Eat a high-fiber diet. Avoid heavy lifting and running. Eliminate the foods and drinks that tend to irritate the bladder, such as alcohol, caffeine, carbonated beverages, spicy foods, sugar, artificial sweeteners, and milk.

10

STRONG BONES FOREVER

•••

- Are you thin, fair-skinned, small-boned?
- Did you have an early menopause?
- Did your mother or grandmother grow notice-ably shorter?
- Do you smoke?
- Do you get very little exercise?
- Have you gone on a lot of low-calorie diets, consumed more than two alcoholic drinks a day, always hated milk?
- Does your family come from the British Isles or northern Europe?

If you answered yes to many of these questions, you are in danger of developing osteoporosis, the brittle bones disease, and you must seriously consider hormone replacement therapy, the *best* way to stop the bone loss that causes it.

Osteoporosis is a bone condition that develops slowly and insidiously after menopause when you no longer produce much estrogen. There are no warning signs, except perhaps for mysterious backaches, and you proba-bly won't know you're about to have trouble until you do—usually in the form of a fracture. By then it's too late to remedy the situation. Osteoporosis is not significantly reversible, so early diagnosis and prevention are extremely important. Preventive efforts must start just after menopause when you'll have a rapid loss of bone mass, because that loss can be slowed, stopped, and perhaps reversed before permanent damage is done.

WHAT CAUSES OSTEOPOROSIS?

If you are a woman with a diminished supply of circulating estrogen, your bones cannot absorb and retain sufficient calcium—*no matter how much calcium you consume*—to keep them at full strength, and so they slowly and inexorably become thinner and thinner. First in the spine and later in the hips and wrists, they lose much of their mass, bulk, and density, diminishing at a rate of about 1 percent a year after age 30 or so. With menopause, the loss accelerates to 2 to 3 percent a year, and in some cases as much as 10 percent, especially in the first seven or eight years when half of the bone loss of a lifetime can occur.

Some women may be starting off with an even bigger problem: According to recent research, they have inherited a gene that inhibits the absorption of calcium into the bone cells, making osteoporosis a much more likely prospect.

YOUR CHANGING BONES

Bones are living tissue that is constantly changing. They store calcium and then release it upon demand when it's needed for life-sustaining functions by other parts of the body. Old bone tissue is continually replaced with new in a process called bone remodeling, so the skeleton that's yours today is certainly not the one that will be yours a few years from now.

Before menopause, there is usually a good balance between the formation of new bone and the resorption of the old, if your diet includes sufficient calcium. But after menopause, resorption overtakes replacement even if you get your quota of calcium and exercise, and so your bones gradually become thinner and weaker.

Bone mass reaches its peak density at about the age of 35. That is when you have as much bone as you are ever going to get. After that, bone tissue and strength begin to decline in everyone, man or woman.

But women start out with a flimsier bone structure than men and so can't afford to lose as much bone before running into serious trouble. Indeed, women are four times as likely to get significant osteoporosis as men, who start out with an average of 30 percent more bone mass. Besides, men don't have menopause. The efficient use of calcium is promoted by the male hormone testosterone, which remains in plentiful supply well into old age. In contrast, women's estrogen loss at menopause leads to accelerated bone loss for about seven years before the rate slows down. A woman who lives long enough runs the risk of losing as much as 40 to 45 percent of her bones.

Osteoporosis afflicts up to a third of American women over the age of 60 and leads to 1.5 million fractures every year. It is the cause of all those broken hips, fractured wrists, and dowager's humps among the older female population.

Bone loss can never be fully recovered or replaced. Although some new drugs can reverse a small percentage of the damage, at least in the spine, most of the bone that's gone is gone. Since there is no good cure for osteoporosis, if you are a woman who is a likely candidate for serious bone loss, you must prevent it before it begins— or stop it before it progresses any further.

CALCIUM AND EXERCISE ARE NOT ENOUGH

Although women have suffered with osteoporosis since the beginning of history, this condition has only recently become major news and women are constantly bombarded with advice to get exercise and eat more calcium to ward it off.

But that's *not* enough. Exercise and calcium will certainly help, but all the physical activity and calcium supplements in the world won't protect you if you are a prime suspect for brittle bones. They are not substitutes for estrogen. The *most* effective way to prevent or arrest this condition is with hormone replacement plus, of course, adequate calcium and exercise. The next best way is to use one of the new nonhormonal drugs which we will soon discuss.

It's a Lifetime Commitment

If you are at high risk for osteoporosis, you cannot save your bones without estrogen replacement or one of the bone-preserving drugs, no matter how much calcium you consume. Ideally, you should start HRT immediately after your last menstrual period, or at least within three years, and continue it for life. That's because it works only as long as you take it. If you take it for several years and then quit, your bone loss will begin anew at its accelerated postmenopausal rate. In fact, estrogen's protection against osteoporosis has been found to erode by age 75 for women who have taken it for less than seven years early in menopause. And stopping HRT for more than five years eliminates most of its protection.

In other words, the longer you use estrogen, the greater its beneficial effect on your skeleton. If you start taking it at menopause, you need to continue it for at least 15 to 20 years to be protected when you are elderly.

To bolster this argument, a study reported in 1995 of 9,500 women over 65 concludes that women who began taking estrogen within five years of menopause and continued for the rest of their lives substantially decreased their risk of almost all fractures. They showed a 50 percent reduction in the risk of all nonspinal fractures and a 71 percent decrease in the risk of broken hips and wrists. On the other hand, those who stopped taking estrogen, even if they had taken it for more than 10 years, showed no significant decrease in the risk of fractures.

Accelerated bone loss starts at menopause, no matter what age you have it. That's why women who lose their ovarian function early—say, at 35 rather than 50—are especially vulnerable to major bone loss, and even more so if they also fit into the high-risk category. Their 15 extra years without estrogen give them more time to develop osteoporosis, and many of them start showing signs of it even before they are out of their 50s.

Worse than that, women whose menopause does not occur spontaneously but results from having had their ovaries removed surgically or destroyed by radiation or chemotherapy are even more likely to have bone problems a few years down the road. That's because the abrupt and complete loss of estrogen may have a more severe impact on the rate of bone loss than the more gradual decline that accompanies natural menopause.

A simple hysterectomy—removal of the uterus alone—can cause lower bone mass too, probably because the operation may reduce blood flow to the ovaries, leading to a gradual decline in estrogen levels.

Doesn't Calcium Help?

Of course it does. You require adequate calcium as well as exercise to build strong bones and fill the demands for this vital mineral by other parts of your body. But that is only one part of the answer. Estrogen, while it isn't directly responsible for bone strength, controls the absorption of calcium into the bones and stimulates the production of calcitonin, a hormone that protects bones. When you no longer make much estrogen, your bones quickly start to lose more bulk than they gain, *even* if you are eating your quota of calcium.

This is the bottom line: If you have kept your bones at full strength by eating and exercising properly before menopause and have inherited a sturdy skeleton to start with, a calcium-rich diet and moderate exercise may well be all the protection you need after menopause. You probably have enough bone to last you a lifetime.

But if you haven't, you *must* seriously consider estrogen replacement to stop the unrelenting loss of your bone mass as the years go by.

A CONDITION TO RECKON WITH

Osteoporosis is serious business. It can even be deadly. It affects more than 25 million people in the United States, 80 percent of them women. Although men get it too, osteoporosis is considered a woman's disease because it is primarily the direct result of diminishing female hormones, beginning its nefarious work when estrogen grows scarce.

A Sneeze Can Do It

If osteoporosis gets bad enough, a woman who has it could suffer a broken arm lifting a casserole out of the oven or reaching back to zip up her dress. She could break her foot stepping out of bed or a rib upon sneezing. She could grow noticeably shorter in only a few weeks, develop dowager's hump, have mysterious backaches. Many of the aches and pains of older people result from tiny microfractures and spinal compressions they don't even know they have.

About 350,000 American women a year suffer broken hips because of osteoporosis, with an estimated 30,000 dying of complications and another 100,000 requiring long-term care. One in every three women fractures a hip before the age of 80. One in five American women over 60 with hip fractures dies of complications, making osteoporosis a leading cause of death in the United States. Twelve to 15 percent of those who suffer hip fracture do not survive the six months following the fracture. According to the National Institutes of Health, 50 percent of those who survive will need help with daily activities and 15 to 25 percent must enter long-term care facilities.

Not all women are in serious danger, of course. Those with heavy bones may never be seriously affected because they can lose considerable bone and still have enough to remain strong. And overweight women tend to be at lower risk too because they continue to produce some estrogen from their fat tissue. But thinner women with light frames have less bone to start with and so they have a smaller margin of safety. They need all the help they can get.

Why Can't a Woman Be More Like a Man?

When it comes to bones, men are far superior to women. Men get osteoporosis too, but it develops much later in life for them. Men start out adult life with more massive bones and so they can afford to lose much more bone mass before becoming seriously affected. They also tend to exercise more and eat more calcium-rich foods, especially milk and dairy products, and do not indulge in low-calorie diets that are usually high in protein and deficient in calcium. If men drink heavily, however, they lose some of their edge. Alcohol hinders the absorption of calcium and often replaces nutritious foods.

Even more important, estrogen has the job of stimulating other hormones that control the absorption of calcium by the bones and inhibit its resorption back into the bloodstream. Men, who don't have a menopause, don't lose their testosterone and estrogen as precipitously and quickly as women lose theirs after menopause and so they don't lose bone as fast either.

The incidence of broken bones rises dramatically in women as they get older, surpassing the incidence in men by far. Although at age 45 the risk of wrist fractures is roughly equal between the genders, it then rapidly rises for women so that, in their lifetimes, they suffer 10 times more wrist fractures than men. They have eight times more hip fractures in a lifetime, although at age 45 men are six times more likely to have them.

About 93 percent of all women in the United States who do not take estrogen will have a fracture of the hip, forearm, pelvis, or spine by the age of 85. The risk for men at that age is only a third of that.

WHO GETS OSTEOPOROSIS?

Everybody gets it. It is normal and universal to lose bone as you get older. But severe cases are not normal.

About a quarter of all women get it severely enough to cause them real trouble.

• Osteoporosis is found least often in blacks and most often in whites and Asians. Blacks have been blessed with denser, heavier bones.

• White women of northern European heritage are more likely to develop it than women whose families originated in the southern regions of Europe. A study in Israel, for example, found that the hip fracture rate among Sephardic Jews was only about 60 percent that of Ashkenazi Jews. As a generalization, it is true that the darker your skin, the lower your chances of developing symptomatic osteoporosis.

• Overweight women may continue to convert enough estrogen from adrenal hormones in their fat tissue to help them absorb calcium long after their ovaries have shut down. In general, the greater the body fat, the greater the estrogen production even after menopause.

• There is more osteoporosis among women living in temperate climates than in the tropics.

• Prematurely gray hair may signify a higher risk for osteoporosis, according to recent research which found that people with hair that turned more than 50 percent gray before the age of 40 were over four times more likely to have thin bones and to have a family history of osteoporosis. The researchers speculate that the gene for premature graying could be linked to a gene that helps determine bone mass.

• Women who take thyroid hormones increase their risk of brittle bones. The higher the dose, the greater the bone loss. Estrogen replacement can offset that risk, however.

• Chronic use of steroids in pill or inhaler forms can cause dramatic bone loss. The higher the dose and the longer the use, the greater the loss. Corticosteroid users must be sure to start HRT immediately after menopause.

• Excessive doses of other drugs can also affect the absorption or retention of calcium by the bones. These include some furosemide diuretics, anticonvulsant drugs, sedatives, muscle relaxants, some oral antidiabetic agents, antacids containing aluminum, cholestyramine, bulk-producing therapeutic fiber preparations, and tetracycline antibiotics.

High-Risk Checklist

The following is the long list of increased risk factors for osteroporosis. If many of them apply to you (especially those at the top of the list), you must take immediate measures to prevent or arrest excessive bone loss. This means hormone replacement therapy starting right after menopause.

The *minimum* dosage for prevention of osteoporosis is 0.625 mg of conjugated estrogen a day (or the equivalent dose of other estrogen). It is best taken every day of the month.

Menopause before 40

Family history of osteoporosis

Family origin in British Isles, northern Europe, Asia

Heavy cigarette smoking (one-half pack or more per day)

Loss of height, especially in upper body

Fracture with no known cause

Hyperparathyroid disease

Uremia

Increased cortisone production or previous long-term cortisone ingestion

Vitamin D deficiency

Very fair skin

Small bones

Consumption of more than 5 ounces of alcohol per day

Liver disease

Diet low in calcium

Lactase deficiency

Malabsorption problem

Hyperthyroidism

Underweight

Sedentary lifestyle

Previous high-protein, low-carbohydrate dieting for more than a year in adulthood

GETTING YOUR BONES TESTED

Today you can have the density of your bones tested with sophisticated and reliable screening techniques. Don't bother if you plan to start HRT at menopause because the estrogen will eliminate the problem. But be sure to be tested before you decide *not* to go on hormone therapy.

The best test is called dual-energy X-ray absorpitiometry, better known as DEXA. It accurately measures bone mineral density in the spine, hip, or wrist, takes only a few minutes, and involves only a tiny amount of radiation. But DEXA is expensive and not available everywhere. Other recommended tests include single-energy X-ray absorptiometry (SPA) and radiographic absorptiometry.

A simple and inexpensive test for bone density, but *only* for screening, is the "heel test." This uses ultrasound—high-frequency sound waves—to measure the density of the heel. If it indicates osteoporosis, it should be followed up by more sophisticated testing.

Using these methods, bone loss of only 1 or 2 percent can be detected. Some physicians still use standard X-rays to diagnose osteoporosis, but it doesn't pick up the damage until you have lost 25 to 30 percent of your bone mass, by which time it's too late to do much about it.

CT scans (computerized tomography) with special attachments can also do an excellent job of diagnosing bone loss, but they are rarely used except in special cases because they require at least 9 rads of radiation, three times the amount for a standard chest X-ray.

Two simple urine tests can provide an indication of active bone loss, which can then be followed up by a bone density test. Called NTX and Pylorynx, they work by measuring the amount of breakdown substances excreted in the urine. Although they are not accurate enough for the diagnosis of osteoporosis, they can help in monitoring the effectiveness of bone-building medications.

Lost height is a good rough indication of osteoporosis that is already doing its destructive work. The body is measured from the crown of the head to the pubic bone, then from the pubic bone to the base of the heel. The measurements in normal people are almost always exactly the same for both halves of the body. If, however, the upper body is an inch or more shorter than the lower half, you probably have vertebral compression from osteoporosis.

Serious tooth loss may also be a sign for older women that their bones are thinning. The teeth are anchored in the jawbones and dwindling bone density leads to loosening teeth, according to current research at Tufts University.

WHAT ESTROGEN DOES FOR YOUR BONES

Estrogen replacement in adequate doses will prevent bone loss before it begins, even among high-risk women, *if* it is started immediately after menopause. It will stop osteoporosis from progressing any further, whenever you start it after menopause. By the way, the transdermal patch appears to be just as good for your skeleton as oral estrogen. Vaginal estrogen cream, however, should not be relied on to preserve your bones.

As for progesterone, it has been found to accentuate the effect of estrogen, producing even thicker and stronger bone tissue than estrogen alone.

The results of the few studies where estrogen was given in combination with testosterone show that the male hormone also helps to produce superior bone tissue, which is logical since it is testosterone as well as estrogen that prevents the early onset of osteoporosis in men.

Many studies have shown that the incidence of spine and hip fractures is lower among women on HRT and that bone loss is stopped or prevented. Our own 10-year study reported back in 1979 was the first study usually cited as decisive evidence for these conclusions. In our pioneer research, 168 women were divided into matched pairs. One of each pair took daily estrogen and progesterone for 10 years, while the other received placebos. Of the 51 women still in the study at the end of the 10 years, those who began HRT within three years of menopause increased their bone mass. Those who started more than three years after their last periods and had already lost bone showed no additional loss. All of the women on placebos, however, showed significant loss.

Among other well-controlled clinical studies was an important nine-year, double-blind study in Scotland, by Dr. Robert Lindsay and colleagues. The results showed "a significant reduction in height" among women who were not given estrogen. The women on HRT did not get shorter. Dr. Lindsay has also concluded, in another study in the United States, that a daily dose of at least 0.625 mg of conjugated estrogen (or the equivalent) is needed to prevent bone loss.

In 1984, the advisory panel to the National Institutes of

Health gave a strong endorsement to estrogen for the prevention of osteoporosis. The FDA added its approval in 1986.

Low-Dose Estrogen for Bone Loss

Women on hormone therapy have almost always been started with a daily dose of 0.625 mg a day of conjugated estrogen (or the equivalent), because it has long been considered the minimum amount for the prevention of bone loss. But it has been found that some women can get along on only 0.03 mg, the lowest dose to receive FDA approval for osteoporosis. A study involving 406 postmenopausal women at 29 medical centers found that women who took daily doses of 0.3 mg of Estratab, estrogen synthesized from soy and yams, had significantly less bone loss than women on placebos. On the other hand, they did not do as well as those taking 0.625 mg. A recent study confirms the adequacy of 0.03 mg if it is bolstered by sufficient amounts of vitamin D and calcium.

Do All Women Need HRT?

Of course not. If you've got good strong bones and have no other problems because of estrogen deficiency, you don't need it. It is always best not to take unnecessary medications.

ESTROGEN AND CALCIUM

According to many studies and a prestigious advisory panel to the National Institutes of Health, estrogen replacement is the single most effective way to prevent osteoporosis. It is probably the only way to keep it from becoming a serious problem. Although other measures, which we will describe shortly, can help, they cannot compare in effectiveness to estrogen nor will they prevent the condition in susceptible women.

One important piece of evidence is a study made by Bruce Ettinger, M.D., of Kaiser Permanente in California, that compared the effects of calcium supplements alone to those of estrogen. A group of 83 volunteers in the early years of menopause were divided into three categories; some were given 0.3 mg of conjugated estrogen a day, plus 1,500 mg of calcium; a second group received 0.625 mg of estrogen and *no* calcium. The third group took 1,500 mg of calcium a day and *no* estrogen. Dr. Ettinger found after a year that those on minimal estrogen plus calcium did not lose bone; those on 0.625 mg of estrogen without calcium also lost no bone; the women on 1,500 mg of calcium without estrogen lost a significant amount of bone.

Dr. Ettinger's 1993 study at Kaiser Permanente showed that once women stopped taking estrogen, bone loss resumed once more.

THE CASE FOR CALCIUM

Most women do not consume enough calcium, certainly not enough to start off with strong bones at the age of 35 and nowhere near enough to end up with a sturdy skeleton at 65 or 70. The average American woman at midlife gets only 400 or 500 mg of calcium in her diet. That's about half the recommended daily allowance of 1,000 mg for premenopausal women and less than that of the 1,500 mg dose recommended for those past menopause.

Why You Need More Calcium

Do you get enough calcium every day? Have you stopped drinking milk under the misconception that you don't need it after you've grown up? Do you worry so much about cholesterol and your weight that you have eliminated some of the foods that are best for you? If you are a typical American woman, it is most unlikely that you get enough calcium, especially since you are probably perennially on a diet. It is *impossible* to get enough of this mineral from food when you eat very few calories.

The important fact to remember is that, when there is not enough calcium available from the food you eat, your body will take what it needs right out of your skeleton. Young women should eat sufficient calcium because it is vital to start out with the maximum allotment of bone. Older women should be especially conscious of calcium consumption because, without enough of the mineral on hand to supply vital body functions, their bones will be plundered to provide it. Besides, their calcium absorption is not as efficient as it used to be.

That is why calcium supplements are essential for virtually everyone. Before menopause, you need them if you don't drink at least three 8-ounce glasses of milk (skim milk contains as much calcium as whole milk, no fat, and only 80 calories) or their equivalent a day. The same applies if you are on HRT after menopause. But if you don't take estrogen, you need supplements unless you consume at least *five* glasses of milk or their equivalent daily.

Your Calcium Quota

- Before menopause, you require a minimum of 1,000 mg of calcium a day in food and/or supplements.

- If you have had menopause *and* take estrogen, you also require at least 1,000 mg.

- If you have had menopause and do *not* take estrogen, you need a minimum of 1,500 mg a day.

Important Facts About Calcium

• Calcium is best absorbed if it is taken throughout the day, rather than all at once. So take several daily doses or take it in time-release capsules. It is also absorbed better if it is taken with meals or a snack when the stomach's production of hydrochloric acid is at its peak. Taking it on an empty stomach could be irritating.

• Don't go overboard with calcium supplements. It causes constipation in some people and excessive amounts may interfere with the body's ability to absorb iron and zinc. Don't take more than 600 mg of elemental calcium at any one time, or over 2,000 a day, to diminish the possibility of gastric reactions. Besides, you can only absorb that much at a time and the rest will be excreted.

• Drink plenty of water every day. This is good for many reasons but, in this case, it helps in the absorption of calcium.

• Antacids that are aluminum derivatives (alhydroxides) take calcium *out* of the body. Check the labels for these ingredients if you habitually take them, and don't use them as a calcium source.

• Regular use of laxatives can interfere with calcium absorption.

• A very high-fiber diet, beneficial in many other ways, can reduce your absorption of calcium. A large consumption of fiber inhibits the absorption of valuable nutrients, including calcium, because the food passes through your body so quickly. For the same reason, don't take calcium supplements at the same time as bulk-forming preparations.

• Don't take your supplements together with iron supplements. Calcium interferes with absorption of iron.

• Do not rely on leafy green vegetables for your major source of calcium. We will explain why below.

• Your bones can only get as thick and dense as your genes have preordained them to become. While you certainly need enough calcium to build them to their optimum size and strength by age 35 or so, they can only reach their own genetic potential. When you have reached your daily threshold for calcium, taking more does no good since you will only excrete the excess.

• Taking lots of calcium, according to recent studies, rarely promotes kidney stones as we used to think it did. Instead it sometimes helps to prevent them.

• Avoid the calcium-enriched "juice drinks," which are 90 percent sugar and water and only 10 percent juice. A more nutritious option is fortified juice that provides 300 mg of calcium in an 8-ounce serving.

Good Food Sources of Calcium

We should all eat foods rich in calcium, especially after menopause. If you don't like your milk straight, eat cheese, yogurt, or other milk products instead, but be sure to eat enough of them. Not all dairy products are good calcium sources. Butter, cream cheese, and cream are high in fat but low in calcium content. If you're allergic to milk, try Lactaid calcium-fortified nonfat milk.

Check the calcium content of the top food sources listed here, add up what you typically eat in a day, and make sure you get at least 1,500 mg if you don't take estrogen and 1,000 mg if you do. If you can't possibly manage to get that much in your diet, then you must take calcium supplements. Include sardines or other soft-boned fish such as canned salmon (eat the bones!) and leafy green vegetables.

Caution: Many leafy greens, including spinach, beet greens, and Swiss chard, are actually calcium *blockers.* They contain oxalic acid, which inhibits the body's absorption of calcium and other nutrients. So, although they are full of this valuable mineral, you won't get the entire benefit of it and, in fact, when you eat them with milk or other calcium sources, you may be blocked from getting all of the benefit of *their* calcium as well.

A diet high in fat will also decrease the amount of calcium you will absorb, as will large doses of zinc or mega-doses of vitamin A.

Although many other foods, from sesame seeds to oysters, contain calcium, let's face it: It is virtually impossible to get your daily allotment of 1,000 to 1,500 mg in your diet without consuming considerable amounts of milk or milk products. If you don't drink enough milk or eat enough dairy products, you need calcium supplements to bring the numbers up. Your body does not care where the mineral comes from.

High-Calcium Food Sources

Food	Portion	Calcium
Milk, whole	1 cup	288 mg
Milk, skim	1 cup	296 mg
Yogurt, whole milk	1 cup	274 mg
Yogurt, skim	1 cup	452 mg
Swiss cheese	1 ounce	260 mg
Sardines, canned, with bones	8 medium	354 mg

Food	Portion	Calcium
Salmon, canned, with bones	3 ounces	160 mg
Tofu	4 ounces	152 mg
Collards	½ cup	179 mg
Dandelion greens	½ cup	140 mg
Kale	½ cup	103 mg
Broccoli	½ cup	50 mg
Lima beans	½ cup	81 mg
Almonds, shelled	½ cup	168 mg
Figs, dried	5 medium	126 mg

Choosing a Calcium Supplement

In general, what you should look for in a supplement is a high percentage of calcium, low cost, and lack of toxic contaminants. All supplements are compounds of calcium and other elements. What's important for you to know is the bioavailability of the calcium, so read the label on the back of the bottle and look for the amount of *elemental calcium* per tablet. That's the amount that's available for absorption. With less concentrated sources you must take more pills a day in order to end up with the same total amount of calcium.

Many of the supplements are made from calcium carbonate, which is easily absorbed, contains the highest amount of elemental calcium per tablet, and is the cheapest. However, it sometimes causes gassiness or constipation. Take it with a little food.

Tricalcium phosphate supplements provide the same amount of calcium but without the gassy side effects.

Calcium citrate is the most readily absorbed form of calcium although it contains only about half as much bioavailable elemental calcium per tablet as calcium carbonate. As a result, you'll have to swallow more calcium citrate to fulfill your daily requirements. It is also more expensive. The kind found in calcium-fortified orange juice, it's a good choice for people with achlorhydria, or decreased stomach acid, a common condition in older people.

Many women like to take oyster shell calcium because it is natural, like sardines, and it is a perfectly good source of calcium carbonate, although no better than others and more expensive. So are some antacids such as Tums-Ex and Calcium Rich Rolaids. The problem here is that you need more tablets a day to meet your requirements. Remember to avoid using the antacids that are aluminum derivatives (alhydroxides) because they *remove* calcium from the body.

Do not take bonemeal or dolomite as a source of calcium because they may be contaminated with significant amounts of lead or other toxic metals. Besides, they may not be adequately absorbed by the body.

Test Your Calcium Tablets

Some brands of calcium tablets do not disintegrate quickly enough in the stomach to ensure absorption. Try dropping one of your tablets in a saucer and covering it with white vinegar. If it doesn't dissolve into powder within half an hour, try another brand.

THE ROLE OF VITAMIN D

Vitamin D is critical to the absorption of calcium and also regulates bone metabolism. So obviously you need it. But don't overdo it. Most people get plenty of D from sunlight and diet, especially since milk is fortified with it and calcium tablets often include it. So unless you are very old, never get out of doors, or eat poorly, don't worry about it.

If you do add vitamin D to your regime, take only a minimal amount—250 international units a day is plenty most of the year and 400 IU in the winter. If you are over 65, says the *Harvard Medical School Health Letter,* you may need a little more, perhaps 800 IU a day, because aging reduces the capacity of the skin to use sunlight for vitamin D. But more can be toxic. Check out your calcium supplements. If they include vitamin D, add up the total you'll be getting in a day and be sure you aren't taking too much.

You really don't need vitamin D supplements in any case if you take HRT, because estrogen increases the production and absorption of the vitamin (in its activated form of calcitriol). Just be sure you get adequate calcium and exercise in addition to your estrogen.

THREATS TO YOUR BONES

Salt, Caffeine, and Alcohol

A high intake of salt increases the excretion of calcium into the urine, which means less is retained by the bones. The same has been thought to be true of caffeine in coffee, tea, and soft drinks, although recent research indicates there may be no connection. As for alcohol, heavy drinkers lose bone at a faster rate than light drinkers and abstainers, probably because alcohol can also inhibit calcium retention.

Smoking

Smoking puts you into one of the highest risk groups for osteoporosis, partly because it can cause an earlier menopause than you were genetically programmed to have, giving you more years to lose bone mass, and partly because it reduces ovarian function and your production of estrogen and progesterone. It can even cancel out the protection provided by HRT. Bone loss is about twice as rapid among thin postmenopausal women who are heavy smokers as among thin postmenopausal women who don't smoke.

Diuretics

Long-term use of thiazide diuretics, commonly used to treat hypertension, has been found to provide some degree of protection against osteoporosis and its resulting high rate of hip fractures among older women. The thiazides do their job only when they are taken in pure form and not in combination with other drugs.

High-Protein Diets

If you want to lose weight in a hurry, a high-protein diet is fine for a week or so, but never longer because it isn't healthy. One reason is that it leads to acidosis. Even moderate acidosis increases the excretion of calcium and can cause osteoporosis over a long enough time. This makes women who persistently follow bizarre diets that lack the normal balance of foods more likely to develop brittle bones. There is also some evidence that excessive consumption of animal protein blocks calcium absorption and, in fact, vegetarians tend to have denser bones than meat eaters unless they are too thin.

Tamoxifen (Nolvadex)

Tamoxifen, a SERM or "selective estrogen-receptor modulator," was created to counteract estrogen's ability to accelerate the growth of breast tumors. It works to prevent tumors in high-risk women and as a treatment for early-stage breast cancer, cutting nearly in half the chance of the cancer occurring in the other breast.

Whether it actually prevents new cases of breast cancer remains a question. Two recently reported European trials, one in Italy, the other in the United Kingdom, showed no protective effect for the drug. A U.S. study of 13,000 healthy women on tamoxifen or placebo, on the other hand, found fewer cancers in the group taking tamoxifen.

Like most potent drugs, tamoxifen has significant side effects. The good news is that it protects the bones from losing their density after menopause for as long as it is used. Not so good news is that it raises the risk of uterine cancer, blood clots, and cataracts, and increases menopausal symptoms such as hot flashes and vaginal dryness.

ALTERNATIVE TREATMENTS FOR FRAGILE BONES

If you take HRT early enough, you won't have to worry about osteoporosis. Estrogen prevents bone loss or stops it in its tracks at whatever stage it has reached. But for the women with breast cancer who have been advised not to take estrogen and women who are suffering from already fragile bones, several alternative treatments are now available, all of them designed to help rebuild lost bone tissue. None of them works as well as estrogen.

Although estrogen replacement remains the gold standard and is the most effective treatment for osteoporosis, doing a better job of arresting and restoring bone mass, two new drugs offer excellent alternatives for women who need prevention of osteoporosis but can't or won't take hormones. Neither Fosamax and Evista, which we will discuss below, are substitutes for estrogen, which has been studied for more than half a century and, in addition to its many proven benefits, is almost 100 percent more effective in the prevention of osteoporosis. Besides, the new drugs have not been around very long and their long-term effects remain unknown. But, for the right women, they do provide options which were not available a few years ago. Where there was only estrogen for osteoporosis, now there is a choice. And there are even more alternative treatments on the way.

Fosamax (Alendronate)

Although not as effective as estrogen, Fosamax (alendronate) is the next best treatment for women with advanced osteoporosis. It can slow bone loss and build bone mass, helping to prevent further fractures. Taken orally, it has been found to reduce hip fractures by 56 percent and spine fractures by 49 percent in high-risk women.

The downside is that Fosamax is hard to absorb and can cause inflammation of the esophagus, heartburn, chest pain, and indigestion. To avoid the gastrointestinal side effects, it must be taken with at least 8 ounces of plain water on an empty stomach first thing in the morning, followed by a half-hour sitting or standing upright with no food or drink. Unlike estrogen, Fosamax works only on your bones and does not help other parts of your body such as your heart, skin, vagina, bladder, and brain.

Taking a bone-building drug in combination with estrogen is probably the best response to a diagnosis of severe osteoporosis because each of them potentiates the other's effects on the bones. Data presented at the European Congress of Osteoporosis in Berlin in 1998 indicates that women taking the combination of HRT *and* Fosamax together show significantly larger increases in bone density at the spine and the hip than those on either therapy alone.

Evista (Raloxifene)

This, like tamoxifen, is one of a new class of drugs called a "selective estrogen-receptor modulator" or SERM. Approved in 1998 by the FDA, it has been called a "designer estrogen," but in fact it is not a hormone and cannot be considered a valid substitute for estrogen. It was created to block the effects of estrogen in certain parts of the body where excessive estrogen may be harmful, such as the breasts and the uterus, and at the same time to fight osteoporosis. It has been found to increase bone density in the spine and hip and reduce the risk of spinal fractures. The results of an international study reported in 1999 showed that, at least short term, it reduces the risk of breast cancer, probably by occupying the same molecular receptor sites as the estrogen molecule on the surface of cells. Because of its selectivity, it is already the first line of treatment for women with osteoporosis who are also at high risk for breast cancer.

Added features are that it does not have gastrointestinal side effects, it does not increase the risk of endometrial cancer, at least over a period of 40 months, and it improves total cholesterol levels. It does not, however, raise HDL, the beneficial cholesterol, as estrogen does. It is too early to know if it affects brain function.

On the downside, this drug increases the risk of blood clots and makes a dry vagina even worse. What's more, it can induce severe hot flashes, even among women who haven't had them for years.

Nor does Evista do as good a job on rebuilding bones as either estrogen or Fosamax. Clinical trials involving 12,000 women in 25 countries for up to 2 years showed that women who took raloxifene increased bone mass by 2 to 3 percent in the hip, spine, and neck, as compared to women who took a placebo. In contrast, women who take estrogen often gain up to twice that amount in bone density, especially in the spine.

In cases of severe osteoporosis, a combination of Evista and estrogen has been found to be the best formula because they potentiate each other's effectiveness. And some specialists now prescribe Evista and Fosamax together for maximum effect.

Sodium Fluoride

People in high-fluoride areas show a greater average bone density (and tooth retention) than those residing in areas with low amounts in their drinking water. And a study from Finland suggests that a small amount of fluoride in the drinking water can lower the number of hip fractures in older people by about a third.

So sodium fluoride has long been thought to be a logical treatment for bones made brittle by osteoporosis. Until recently, however, it didn't work out that way. Although it produced new bone, that bone proved to be more brittle than ever and, at the same time, it caused a vast array of distressing side effects.

Calcitonin-Salmon (Miacalcin)

Approved for the treatment of osteoporosis in 1995, calcitonin-salmon is a synthetic form of a hormone produced by the thyroid. Taken by nasal spray in combination with calcium, it can increase bone density in the spine. Another option for women who refuse to take or can't take estrogen, it can have uncomfortable side effects such as nasal irritation or inflammation and headaches.

Parathyroid Hormone

Still considered an experimental drug, parathyroid hormone, which helps govern calcium absorption, has been found to prevent bone loss in young women who are severely estrogen-deficient, according to research at Massachusetts General Hospital reported in 1998. Also, scientists at the University of California at San Francisco studied postmenopausal women taking a corticosteroid such as prednisone, which weakens bones by slowing the absorption of calcium from food and suppressing bone-making cells. They found that treating them with daily injections of parathyroid hormone plus estrogen, vitamin D, and calcium supplements actually fostered bone growth dramatically by increasing the number of bone-building cells called osteoblasts. Ongoing trials of the effect of this hormone on the usual cases of post-menopausal osteoporosis are also expected to produce good results.

Keep in mind, however, that the dosages of parathyroid hormone must be very carefully controlled. If not, it can be dangerous—too much causes severe bone loss, just the opposite of what you want.

Etidronate

Etidronate, marketed under the brand name Didronel for yet another bone disease, can increase bone mass and has been reported to cut the incidence of fractures of the spine in half for women who already have debilitating osteoporosis. But etidronate has not yet been approved for this use by the FDA and its long-term effects have not been determined.

Calcitriol

Yet another medication for breast cancer patients who suffer badly from osteoporosis but can't take HRT, calcitriol is a synthetic form of vitamin D. Still experimental, it is taken along with calcium supplements and has been found in trials to reduce spinal fractures.

Risedronate (Actonel)

Risedronate is another bone-building drug that at this writing is about to be approved by the FDA for marketing as an osteoporosis remedy. It, like alendronate, is a potent biphosphonate, a compound that works only on bone tissue and does not affect—so far as is known to date—any other part of the body either for good or for bad. It inhibits bone breakdown and has been shown to increase bone density, thereby reducing the risk of fractures.

Risedronate (Actonel) differs from alendronate (Fosamax) in one important way and that is that it does not seem to cause the same gastrointestinal problems. It too must be taken first thing in the morning on an empty stomach and must not be diluted by food for at least half an hour, but does not require an upright position and probably will not upset the stomach or irritate the esophagus.

In a study at the University of California at San Francisco reported in October 1999, researchers studied 2,458 postmenopausal women under the age of 85 who had suffered at least one spinal fracture prior to the study. The women were randomly assigned to receive risedronate oral tablets or a placebo for three years. The researchers found that those on risedronate were about 40 percent less likely to have new fractures of the spine or other bones than those on placebo.

As with the other similar bone-building medications, however, it is still very early in this drug's life and only with time will we know if it is effective and safe over the long term.

And, like other bone-builders, it is not as effective as estrogen, which has been intensely studied over the last 40 years.

CONSUME CALCIUM!

No matter what kind of bone therapy you are on, it is absolutely essential to consume enough calcium from food or supplements. Calcium boosts the effects of all of the treatments and is required for the formation of new bone. But remember, if you already have significant osteoporosis or are a high-risk candidate for it, calcium alone will not do the job without estrogen or another therapy. Don't wait another moment. Consult with your physician now.

HOW EXERCISE HELPS YOUR BONES

Exercise alone will not maintain the integrity of your bones. You need adequate calcium and a plentiful supply of estrogen if you are not going to lose significant bone mass after menopause. You can exercise for hours a day, consume megamilligrams of calcium, and you will still lose density if you are estrogen-deficient.

That doesn't mean you can afford to sit around, however. Exercise does help. Although we can't build much bone anymore—we achieved our peak bone mass at age 35 or so—we can maintain what we've got. The truth is that bones, like muscles, must be used to keep them at their optimum strength. And the physical activity you need must provide the mechanical stress of muscles pulling on bone. Although weight-bearing and antigravitational exercise is the best, strength training is also beneficial.

Bones respond to physical exertion at any age, although this is the time of our lives when most of us exercise less and sit more. But we need exertion more than ever now to keep every part of our bodies in the best possible shape. So make it a routine part of your life to include moderately vigorous weight-bearing activities for at least a half-hour four times a week plus muscle-strengthening workouts at least twice a week. You'll be doing your bones a real service. You will also be building more muscle mass, making you more likely to avoid and survive falls without damage.

Keep in mind, by the way, that the beneficial effects of exercise last only as long as the exercise continues and dissipate very quickly when you fall back into a sedentary lifestyle.

The Right Kind of Exercise

Almost any kind of vigorous exercise makes you more fit, strengthens your heart and lungs, tones up your muscles, and makes you feel mentally alert. But for better bones, it's most important to stress the long bones of the body and the spine and add the force of gravity. For example, jogging, brisk walking, bicycling, dancing, stair climbing. Brisk walking, by the way, is as good as any other form of exercise. Just be sure you walk fast enough to cover three miles in less than an hour.

Add weight lifting to your regimen too. It has been found that postmenopausal women who train intensively on exercise machines twice a week can increase the size and power of their muscles and improve their balance. That can prevent falls, the greatest risk factor for fractures in older women. It can also increase bone density in the hips and spine, the sites of the most serious fractures caused by osteoporosis.

HRT FOR YOUR TEETH

Researchers from Harvard Medical School/Brigham and Women's Hospital in Boston studied more than 42,000 postmenopausal women and found a 24 percent decrease in tooth loss among HRT users. The results of another long-term study of almost 500 women showed that those on HRT for nine or more years retained the most teeth, nearly four more teeth than women who had never used it.

One reason, of course, may be that women who take HRT tend to be those who are especially concerned for their health and take good care of themselves, including their teeth. Another is that estrogen probably helps the bones of the jaws to retain their density and strength, thereby anchoring teeth more securely.

IT'S NEVER TOO LATE

Estrogen will start doing its job of arresting bone loss whenever you start taking it regularly as a supplement after menopause, so it's never too late to help yourself. Even women in their 80s and 90s can benefit from HRT prescribed to stop osteoporosis from advancing further. And they can sometimes get additional help in building more bone from one of the alternative treatments described earlier in this chapter.

This book has not been written to convince you to take HRT if, for some reason, you don't want to do it. Its purpose is to let you know this proven fact: Nothing will preserve your bones like estrogen. If you don't need it, fine. If you do, don't be afraid of it.

11

YOUR SKIN: WILL ESTROGEN KEEP YOU YOUNG FOREVER?

•••

No, estrogen is not the fountain of youth and it won't keep you young forever. It won't stop the clock or change the effects of normal aging or overexposure to the sun on your skin, but it *can* delay the changes that are specifically due to estrogen loss. Because their skin stays thicker, moister, oilier, and more flexible, women who take HRT tend to look younger than their years.

Consider this a fortunate fringe benefit of HRT because we certainly don't recommend taking estrogen for this reason alone. Hormones are drugs, after all, and we still don't know everything there is to know about them. But if you take them for valid reasons, your skin will prosper as a result.

THE NATURAL HISTORY OF SKIN

As the years go by, the skin, the tough protective covering that is the body's largest organ, gradually loses its thickness, moisture content, and lubrication. It becomes dryer, less resilient, and more lax. Its oil production and ability to sweat dwindle along with its blood supply. Meanwhile, the underlying support structure weakens as its subcutaneous fat layer shrinks, muscle tissue loses bulk and firmness, elastin becomes less resilient, and collagen fibers decrease in number and density. The ability of its cells to renew themselves declines until, at age 60, they take twice as long to replace themselves as when you were young.

And that's not all the bad news. The skin gradually loses its protective pigment cells (the reason your skin doesn't tan as readily), the skin gets thinner and the walls of the superficial blood vessels become more fragile (why bruising and broken veins are more common), your healing processes don't work as well as they once did (why injuries take longer to repair themselves), and the skin becomes a less efficient regulator of body temperature (one reason why you feel chilly more easily).

Exposure to the sun, the skin's arch enemy, accelerates the processes of chronological aging by impairing its immune response and destroying oil glands, collagen, and elastic fibers. An estimated 80 percent of all visible signs of aging and 90 percent of skin cancers are caused by the sun.

Smoking speeds up the damage too by constricting the small blood vessels and reducing the supply of oxygen to the skin. Drastic dieting, quick weight changes, and environmental assaults such as extreme temperatures, low humidity, and air pollution also play their parts.

ESTROGEN'S ROLE

Estrogen too plays a significant role in determining how well your skin makes it through the years. Although hormone replacement won't moderate the changes that happen simply because you are getting older or have inflicted damage on your fragile exterior, it can help hold off the changes that are specifically due to estrogen loss.

Estrogen is partially responsible for the distribution of subcutaneous fat, the layer of fat just under the epidermis that provides inner support, firmness, and resilience. It helps to maintain water in the tissues by stimulating the production of hyaluronic acid that holds water and increasing the extracellular moisture content. It encourages oil production and the formation of collagen, the connective tissue that keeps the skin thick and firm.

For all these reasons, your skin shows the effects of the loss of estrogen as it slowly diminishes, especially in the first few years after menopause.

EVERYONE IS DIFFERENT

Some fortunate women inherit wonderful skin that remains fairly firm and smooth in spite of the passing years if they haven't abused it. In general, these are the ones who, aside from having shunned the sun, do not experience a sudden precipitous drop in estrogen at menopause and continue for most of their lives to produce a certain amount of the hormone, mostly now from their adrenal glands and fat cells.

Women who have a late menopause also tend to have better skin than those who lose their estrogen early. Because they have more years of plentiful estrogen that affects their skin as well as the rest of their bodies, they usually have firmer skin even if they don't go on HRT and tend to look younger than their peers. In fact, according to a recent British study, the condition of the skin correlates more closely with how many years you have spent without estrogen than with how old you are.

Women with a few extra pounds usually look younger after menopause too, not only because their extra fat plumps up their skin but also because they usually continue to make some estrogen in their fat tissue.

WHAT HRT CAN DO

For optimal effects on your skin, HRT should be started very soon after menopause because, like the bones, the skin changes most rapidly in the first several years. But whenever you start, you will probably notice some improvement. Although, as we have said, supplemental estrogen can't change the effects of genetic aging or sun damage, it can help delay the changes due to estrogen loss and improve your skin by adding fat, moisture, oil, and collagen.

The additional subcutaneous fat stimulated by estrogen makes the skin a little tighter, while the increased oil production prevents it from drying out as much as it otherwise would. The ability to retain more collagen, at the same time, makes the skin thicker and firmer. In fact, some British researchers have found that skin is only half as thick in women nearing 60 who do not take estrogen as it is among those who do.

There is, however, an occasional cosmetic side effect for some women when they take estrogen in higher doses. The added hormone sometimes causes increased pigmentation, a slight darkening of the skin here and there, which may not be reversible. This is rare at the usual HRT doses, but talk to your doctor if it happens to you. Your choices are to lower your dose, with your doctor's approval, or to quit the therapy.

SENSIBLE SUGGESTIONS FOR YOUR SKIN

Good skin care can make a big difference in the way your skin looks and lasts. Whether or not you are on HRT, there is much you can do to keep your skin looking younger and fresher.

• First, stay out of the sun. It is your skin's major enemy and its damage cannot be significantly reversed. The more sun you've had, the older your skin will eventually be. When you can't avoid it, use a sunblock or a broad-spectrum sunscreen with an SPF (sun protection factor) of at least 15.

• Try to maintain an environment that is reasonably humid. If you live in a dry climate, a self-sterilizing humidifier is a wise investment.

• Use moisturizer faithfully to reduce the loss of water from the skin's surface by sealing it in. Apply it to damp skin just after a bath or a wash.

• Grease up your skin regularly, again best when it's been hydrated. Petroleum jelly, any kind of oil, vegetable shortening, or oil-based cream or ointment will do. The greasier the better.

• Wash with warm (not hot) water, skipping the soap when possible. If you need more cleansing than that, use a mild nonperfumed soap or a soap substitute. Both soap and hot water tend to eliminate the natural oil barrier that lubricates your skin.

• Drink plenty of fluids, preferably water, which is good for your whole body including your skin.

• Avoid dehydrators such as alcohol, caffeine, diuretics, dry air, and saunas.

• Get plenty of vigorous exercise. Healthy circulation brings more blood to the skin and toned muscles help to round out your contours.

• Use oil-based cosmetics and avoid perfumed skin products.

• Increase your intake of vitamin C.

MORE CREAMS AND LOTIONS

Two topical creams have been developed to help in the battle against fine wrinkles, liver spots, and other skin changes caused by the years and the sun. These are tretinoin (Retin-A), available by prescription, and alpha-hydroxy acids, substances made from natural sources. These acids are now added to many cosmetic creams but are really effective only in higher concentrations that are available only by prescription or in your dermatologist's office.

ESTROGEN AND YOUR BODY HAIR

When you lose estrogen, you tend to lose the hair on your legs, under your arms, and in the pubic area. Sometimes, perhaps 5 or 10 years after menopause, hair starts growing on the face and body where it never grew before and where it is certainly not welcome, especially since it is often dark and coarse.

All this happens because body hair is under the control of your hormones. Some women have hair follicles that are overly sensitive to the androgens (male hormones) that all women normally produce, a tendency that becomes evident after menopause when the androgens become more influential because they are no longer adequately opposed by estrogen. The result is that your hair tends to grow in a more male pattern.

HRT can have a decidedly beneficial effect on unwanted facial and body hair, promptly stopping new growth. An alternative is spironolactone (Aldactone), a mild diuretic that can block the growth of face and body hair for as long as you use it. However, it has not yet been approved for this use by the FDA. Another alternative, of course, is electrolysis.

ESTROGEN AND THE HAIR ON YOUR HEAD

Although the numbers of hairs on their heads diminish gradually for all women as they get older, some women suffer from hereditary hair loss with marked thinning that can't be permanently reversed. If this happens to you, you can blame it on your genes with a little help from your hormones.

HRT doesn't have much effect on thinning hair, although it may thicken it a little and slow down the rate of loss slightly. At the moment, the prescription drug monoxidil (marketed as Rogaine) is the only medication that's been approved by the FDA to treat "male pattern baldness." Applied to the scalp twice a day, every day, it works only as long as it's used, sometimes stimulating some regrowth.

12

Hysterectomies, Oophorectomies, and Instant Menopause

Many women have no idea what happens during a hysterectomy, a surgical procedure that is second only to cesarean delivery as the most common major operation in the United States (more than one out of every three women over 60 has had one). They are confused about what is removed and how this event can affect menopause, their estrogen supply, and the rest of their lives. In this chapter, we discuss this surgery and try to straighten out some common misunderstandings.

WHAT HAPPENS WHEN

When you have a hysterectomy, your uterus including the cervix (or a portion of the cervix) is removed. The cervix is the part of the uterus that forms its base and narrows down to a small opening that meets the vagina. Your ovaries remain intact and undisturbed. So, if you have not already had menopause, you will continue to produce estrogen in your ovaries and you will not have menopause or get any of its typical symptoms at this time. You will have it around the same time you would normally have had it or maybe a little earlier. You won't, however, have any more menstrual periods and you can't get pregnant.

The scenario is very different when your ovaries and fallopian tubes are removed. This surgical procedure is called an oophorectomy and it is often performed during the same operation as a hysterectomy. When you lose your ovaries before you have had menopause, you will have instant and absolute menopause. Without your ovaries, you will secrete no more estrogen (or testosterone, for that matter) except for the small amounts made in the adrenals and fat tissue, and you will have no more menstrual periods. Nor can you get pregnant. And you will have instant (within a day or two of the surgery) symptoms, probably much more severe and long lasting than after a natural menopause because of the very sudden drop in estrogen. In fact, the younger you are at the time of the surgery, the worse the symptoms are likely to be and the longer they will tend to last.

Sometimes a compromise is made and only one of your ovaries is removed. As long as the other is still functioning, none of the above applies because the remaining ovary continues to produce hormones until you have a natural menopause.

If you have already had menopause before this operation, losing your ovaries isn't so dramatic, but it does mean you will no longer have the benefits of the remnants of estrogen and testosterone you may still have been producing. However, you probably won't have hot flashes or the other menopausal symptoms, although occasionally they will make a brief appearance. If that happens, it is because you have continued to make a minimal amount of estrogen from your ovaries, although not enough to stimulate ovulation and menstrual periods.

Very often a hysterectomy (removal of the uterus) and an oophorectomy (removal of the ovaries) are performed at the same time, and most people, physicians included, refer to the whole surgical procedure as a "hysterectomy," although in this case it is much more than that. It is a hysterectomy *and* an oophorectomy. This misuse of terms causes a lot of confusion. It's clear that a new word is needed to describe this double happening.

When only your uterus has been removed, the ovaries do not shrivel and become dysfunctional. They have their own blood supply and continue to function. If the uterus is removed at a relatively young age, however, menopause often arrives earlier than it would have otherwise, sometimes by several years, probably because some of the blood circulation was compromised during the surgery.

The ovaries continue to produce and release eggs every month in the meantime, although these eggs cannot be deposited into a nonexistent uterus for possible fertilization. Instead, they are expelled into the abdominal cavity where they are quickly and harmlessly absorbed.

PELVIC EXAMS ARE STILL ESSENTIAL

Many women assume that, having lost their uterus, there is no reason to have regular pelvic checkups. But routine examinations are still essential. If you still have your ovaries, they and your fallopian tubes must be checked periodically. And, even if you haven't, you should have a vaginal checkup, including a Pap smear, and a breast exam at least once a year. Besides, in the current social climate, sexually transmitted diseases, from often-symptomless chlamydia to AIDS (acquired immune deficiency syndrome), are becoming more and more common among women of all ages and circumstances.

WHY HYSTERECTOMIES?

About a third of all hysterectomies are performed because of large troublesome fibroids, nonmalignant muscular tumors in the uterus that can cause heavy bleeding, pressure on other organs, and sometimes severe pain. However, the majority of women with fibroids have no symptoms and never even know they have them until their gynecologists detect them during a pelvic examination. Fibroids very rarely become malignant. So the thinking today is that benign fibroids, no matter how large they become, must be treated only if the problems they cause become more than you care to live with.

Fibroids can't be cured except by a hysterectomy, although because they are dependent on estrogen for their growth, they will stop growing or even shrink when your estrogen production drops at menopause. When they are removed by myomectomy—a surgical procedure that excises the tumors without removing the uterus—there's no guarantee a new crop won't develop later.

For women who are very close to menopause, another treatment for troublesome fibroids is now available. They can buy time by taking a drug that stops the ovaries from producing estrogen and creates an artificial menopause until it occurs on its own. No longer fueled by estrogen, the fibroids shrink.

By the way, hormone replacement therapy after menopause rarely makes fibroids grow because the estrogen dose is so small, although it may stop them from shrinking. If your fibroids are large and you are afraid the HRT might increase their size, but you really need estrogen's help, you can always try it and see.

Other reasons for hysterectomies include serious infections, endometriosis, adenomyosis, and, of course, can-

cer. Hyperplasia, the overproliferation of the uterine lining, often precipitates surgery too out of fear that it will
become malignant. In some cases, it is even mistaken for
cancer. "Simplex" hyperplasia is rarely a valid reason for
a hysterectomy, however, since it can almost invariably
be successfully treated with progesterone.

Hysterectomies are not the only answer to many other
problems either, and women who express a preference
not to have surgery increase their chances of avoiding
them. Often their doctors then reconsider and suggest
alternative treatments, with younger physicians with
recent training less likely to recommend the operation
than older doctors.

DO YOU STILL HAVE OVARIES?

It's important to know whether you have had a hysterectomy alone or an oophorectomy as well. In other words,
whether you possess one or both of your ovaries. Many
women have no idea whether they do or don't and usually assume that "everything" has been removed. The
women whose ovaries are still intact after a hysterectomy
before menopause are often very surprised years later
when their estrogen production diminishes and they start
having menopausal symptoms.

With your ovaries (or one ovary), you can expect to
have menopause around the time when you would normally have had it, or perhaps a little earlier, complete
with the typical menopausal symptoms.

Aside from avoiding a big surprise when you start
having hot flashes long after a hysterectomy, there's
another good reason for knowing whether your ovaries
have been removed. When you go to a new physician,
you should be able to give a complete medical history so
the doctor can be alert for problems such as cysts or
enlargement or infection of the ovaries.

If you don't know your internal status, ask your present or former physician to check the records or request that the hospital look into its surgical reports. Failing that, your new doctor can use ultrasound to see whether your ovaries are still there. An FSH test, if you are younger than the usual age for menopause, is another detection technique. If your FSH level is low, you still have functioning ovaries.

MAKING A DECISION ABOUT YOUR OVARIES

It usually goes like this: If you are over 40 or 45, your ovaries are removed along with your uterus when you have a hysterectomy because, although they are perfectly healthy, the physician decides you no longer need them, or won't for very long. You are either fast approaching menopause or have already passed it. So, it is suggested, why not eliminate the possibility of future ovarian cancer, a deadly disease with no early warning signs?

But on the other side of the argument, the incidence of ovarian cancer is very low, only about 2 percent. This risk must be weighed against the dramatic effects of losing all of your ovarian function.

You are the one who must decide whether to have your ovaries removed if they are found to be healthy during a hysterectomy, at whatever age you are. It is up to *you* if you wish to take a chance on getting this rare cancer.

There are good arguments on both sides of this debate. Many specialists feel it's better to remove healthy ovaries if you have already had menopause, figuring they are not much use to you anymore. But even after menopause your ovaries continue to turn out *some* estrogen and androgens, sometimes for years, with some women making significant amounts for 10 or 20 years after menopause. This estrogen protects your arteries, your bones, your skin, and your vagina. So you must weigh the benefits against the risks.

Removing healthy ovaries *before* menopause while they are still producing large amounts of estrogen is yet another question. Even at 45 or 50, you may have years to go before menopause. So think about it carefully. To put an end to your major estrogen supply, especially in this abrupt manner, is a serious step because of the degenerative changes it will initiate throughout your body if you don't promptly take hormone replacement therapy.

If you are willing to take the chance that your ovaries will remain healthy—and those of us who don't have hysterectomies *do* take that chance—then you may decide to keep them. Consider the gynecologist's recommendation, get a second opinion, and remember you have an option.

CHECK YOUR FSH

One way to help you make the decision about an oophorectomy is to have your FSH level tested (see Chapter 7). If your FSH is elevated, you will probably have menopause within a year or so. If it is not elevated, you may have years of good estrogen production to go. Ask your female relatives when they had menopause. If, for example, your mother had hers at 58 and you are now 46, you may decide that the possibility of 12 more years of estrogen outweighs the small risk of eventual ovarian problems.

No matter what you decide, however, you should give the surgeon your written permission to remove your ovaries during the procedure if they are found to be diseased. Without that permission, you may face a second operation within a few weeks.

IS HRT NECESSARY?

Hormone replacement therapy is not necessary after having had your ovaries removed before menopause, but it certainly is recommended because it makes life a lot easier. You are likely to have very severe symptoms without it. That's why few women fail to take it and few doctors refuse to prescribe it. Today, it's a rare woman who cannot take it safely.

The other major disadvantage of losing your ovaries before their time is that you now have extra years to live without estrogen's benefits, more time to develop the consequences of an estrogen deficiency—including osteoporosis, sexual difficulties, and a significantly higher risk of heart disease. With HRT you can avoid all of them.

Hormone therapy is usually continued for at least five years after the surgery—this is considered short term—or until you wish to end it. Be sure to stop gradually if you decide to quit, or you may find yourself having the same symptoms all over again. Ovarian cancer, by the way, does not necessarily rule out the use of HRT.

Obviously, if you no longer have a uterus to protect, you need not take progesterone now.

If you cannot take estrogen, then you must cope with the withdrawal symptoms such as hot flashes and atrophic body changes in alternative ways. See Chapter 6 for suggestions.

13

DOCTOR, IS THIS NORMAL?

··

It is an excellent idea to know your body well enough to notice whether anything that's happening is different or perhaps abnormal. During perimenopause and for a few years after menopause, that's sometimes hard to do because your body is changing and you may not know what's normal and what's not.

That's why the more information you have about menopause, the better. This is a time when women tend to become concerned about their health, not only because of the physical changes, erratic periods, and strange sensations, but because, for them, menstruation has always symbolized good feminine health.

For many reasons, it is important to have regular checkups by a competent and knowledgeable physician, and to report to that physician whenever you have an indication that something is wrong or even different.

HEAVY PERIODS: GO TO YOUR DOCTOR

Women in perimenopause often have very copious menstrual periods, perhaps accompanied by clots, almost like minor hemorrhages. Is this normal? Yes. Should it be ignored? No.

Although the heavy flow is almost surely due to hormonal changes, there is always a small possibility that it is not, especially since this is the most common time for the uterine lining to thicken abnormally into hyperplasia, a condition that must not be neglected.

The status of your endometrium can easily be evaluated and treated by your physician. If hyperplasia has developed, two or three months of treatment with progesterone will stimulate the uterus to shed that overproliferated lining. If your periods return to normal, you will know the heavy bleeding occurred because you were not ovulating or producing your own progesterone.

If, however, the periods don't become normal, then the bleeding must be considered abnormal and further investigation is essential.

UNSCHEDULED BLEEDING: GO TO YOUR DOCTOR

If you have bleeding or spotting *at any time* other than during your periods or the miniperiods stimulated by HRT (see Chapter 7), again consider it abnormal and report it to your doctor promptly.

Unscheduled bleeding may be caused by hyperplasia, polyps (small benign growths), fibroids (the most common cause of unplanned bleeding), or some other problem including cancer. Occasionally, a woman who is not taking estrogen will have spotting because of atrophic vaginitis, when the vaginal lining becomes so thin, raw, and irritable that it bleeds very easily, especially after intercourse.

After your menstrual periods have stopped for about six months, any new bleeding (except for regular HRT-induced miniperiods) means you must go to your doctor for another examination to be sure all is well. That is advisable although it would be quite possible and normal for your periods to make an appearance again even after so many months. Check with your doctor, too, if you have these periods at less than three-week intervals.

TESTING YOUR ENDOMETRIUM

There are several ways your gynecologist can evaluate the health of your uterine lining. Here are the usual procedures.

Pap smear. In this quick screening test, a sample of cells from the lower end of the cervix (the bottom section of the uterus) and the upper vagina are scraped or brushed off, smeared on a glass slide, and sent to a laboratory for close examination under a microscope. A Pap smear may give you a sense of security when the results of the test are negative, but it is a false security because the smear tests only cervical and vaginal cells. It is *not* a reliable test of the endometrium.

Progesterone challenge test. To test the endometrium before menopause, you are given oral progesterone (and no estrogen), usually in doses of 10 mg a day for seven days for one or two consecutive months. If the progesterone regulates perimenopausal periods, making them become regular and normal in both flow and timing, this is an excellent indication that your uterine lining is normal.

If you've already had menopause and you don't have any vaginal bleeding after taking 10 mg a day of oral progesterone for 12 days, it is unlikely that you have an overly thickened lining or, in other words, hyperplasia. If you do bleed and an endometrial biopsy then shows you have simple hyperplasia, treatment with progesterone for two or three months will almost invariably reverse it. If you have atypical cells (complex hyperplasia), you need further evaluation, probably by D&C.

Endometrial biopsy. An office procedure, the biopsy has almost completely replaced the D&C (dilatation and curettage), once the only way to get a sample of the endometrium. A slender catheter or pipelle is inserted into your vagina and passed through the cervix into your uterus. Then suction is used to trap endometrial cells for a microscopic examination by a pathologist, who looks for abnormal or excessive numbers of cells. A procedure that takes only a couple of minutes, the biopsy is usually painless, although you may experience some minor cramping. You can minimize the cramping by taking two antiprostaglandin tablets, such as Advil or Anaprox, an hour or two beforehand.

Transvaginal ultrasound. This noninvasive technique can be an excellent screening method for measuring the thickness of the endometrium, although it does not retrieve cells for microscopic examination. If the endometrium has not overproliferated and therefore is thin, you are pronounced safe from hyperplasia. If it is thick, it must be further investigated by endometrial biopsy.

Dilatation and curettage (D&C). This is a minor 15-minute operation usually performed in the hospital under general anesthesia. It is never done routinely, but as the next step when abnormal cells have been detected in the tissue retrieved by biopsy. Sometimes, too, a D&C is required when the uterus is enlarged, bleeding is very heavy or persistent, the cervix is too narrow to admit the pipelle, polyps are suspected, or too little tissue can be taken by aspiration. The cervix is dilated and a curette is used to scrape and remove the uterine lining. Samples of the tissue are sent to a laboratory for examination.

FINDING THE RIGHT DOCTOR

Most women spend more time and energy shopping for a new car or buying a coat than they do looking for a doctor. But choosing the right doctor is far more important than almost any other decision you'll ever need to make. There may come a critical moment when your future is in that person's hands, and that is no time to discover you haven't made the right choice. If you are typical, you usually see a physician only when you have a problem and, then, you may be strangers to one another. You cannot be sure you're getting the best treatment if you have not established a relationship or had an opportunity to check out this person's credentials.

Most women find new physicians through the recommendation of friends or relatives. If your friends or relatives are the kind of people who investigate their choices thoroughly, fine. But usually *they* found the doctor through their next-door neighbor's cousin who was influenced by her hairdresser. It is safer not to rely solely on such references. This is an important decision.

Shop around for a physician, just as you would for a car. It is usually best to choose one recommended by another doctor whom you trust. Ask questions, get opinions from patients, poll your friends, check credentials and affiliations in reference books found in your public library. Make sure your possible choice graduated from a reputable medical school and performed a residency at a major hospital. An added assurance of quality is board certification; in the case of a gynecologist, she or he should be board-certified in obstetrics and gynecology. Another route is to call or write the chief of medicine at the best hospital in your area and ask for a recommendation. You may also be able to investigate physicians through public interest groups in your community. Consumer organizations in many states have prepared consumers' guides to doctors.

When you have a recommendation, your decision should still await further investigation. Make sure the physician has privileges to practice at a hospital that is convenient, competent, and reputable. Then consider interviewing the doctor before becoming a patient. This person may be an excellent physician but poor in human relations. You should find someone who provides what you need. Some women want to be told what to do, while others want to share in the decision making of their treatment. The relationship must be a comfortable one that satisfies you both intellectually and emotionally.

You must be able to talk to your doctor, to confide and discuss the most delicate subjects. You must feel you are not being rushed out of the office before you have asked all of the questions you want to ask and that you have received satisfactory answers. You need a good listener, neither too authoritative nor casual, who won't be affronted by naive questions or strong opinions. This is especially important at menopause because the physician may have views about it that do not match yours. He or she may have gone through menopause before with hundreds of patients, but *you* haven't.

After you have chosen a new doctor, remember that you are not married to this person and you do not require a divorce if the match doesn't work out. If you do not think you are getting the best care or if there is a communication problem, don't go back. Conduct a new search and find someone who suits you better.

DO YOU NEED A GYNECOLOGIST?

Every woman, especially after the age of 40, should have a complete pelvic examination at least once a year and every six months if she is on medication such as hormone replacement. Many general doctors and internists consider the female reproductive system part of their expertise and routinely perform their own pelvic exams. If they encounter a problem they cannot handle, they will (or should) send you to a gynecologist.

In general, however, it is best to have a family doctor

or internist whom you see once a year for a physical checkup *and* a gynecologist whom you see at least once a year for a pelvic examination, whether or not you think you have a problem. A gynecologist is a physician with advanced training in women's health and is a specialist in the female reproductive system. This specialist sees many more cases of hyperplasia, vaginal infections, sexual problems, and breast lumps, and is usually much more knowledgeable about menopause, menopausal symptoms, atrophic vaginas, and HRT. Most important, he or she is much more likely than an internist to have kept up with the most recent developments in this sophisticated and constantly changing field.

In some cases, your internist or gynecologist may recommend a consultation with a reproductive endocrinologist, a physician who has first trained in internal medicine or gynecology and has then taken advanced training in female hormones. You will never see an endocrinologist routinely, but only when there is a question of hormonal dysfunction. If your doctor does not recommend a consultation but you are having great difficulties, have strong doubts about how your case has been handled, or think you need the opinion of a hormone specialist, suggest it yourself or arrange to see this person on your own.

14

FIGHT BACK! IT'S YOUR OWN BODY!

•••

In this book, we have tried to answer all of your questions about menopause and hormone replacement therapy, to give you the facts and the fictions, the history and the science, the trade-offs and the alternatives, so you can make your own decision about what's going on inside of you and what you want to do about it. You are likely to live another 30, 40, or even 50 years beyond menopause, and what you choose to do can make a remarkable difference on the quality of those years. In fact, this is one of the most important health decisions you will ever make.

NO NEED TO SUFFER

Menopause is not a disease and so it need not be cured. It is a natural and normal physiological phase of life. But when it becomes a difficult phase, it makes no sense not to look for help. If you are having problems because of menopausal symptoms or physical changes, fight back! Refuse to accept them unnecessarily. It's your body, you are the one who must live with it, and you should take charge of it when you can.

With menopausal problems as with any other physical problems, learn everything you can about them. Find out what all your options are. Decide if you need help, and if you do, go get it. Try the nonmedical alternatives first if you like and, if they don't work for you, go further.

You can prepare for menopause by taking care of your body, eating the right foods, getting enough exercise, following good living habits, and maintaining emotional health. But sometimes, no matter how prepared you are, how healthy, how well conditioned, how sane and occupied and fulfilled you've been, how many vitamins, minerals, herbs, and containers of yogurt you've consumed, you are still going to have disabling hot flashes, palpitations, tingling fingers, or sleepless nights. Sometimes, no matter how prepared you are, you are still going to develop brittle bones that break for no good reason, arteries that get rigid and clogged, or a vagina that gradually becomes physically incapable of sexual intercourse.

Sometimes you need help to overcome problems— and you have a right to have it. In only the past few years, times and opinions have changed dramatically as scientific knowledge about women's health has increased and attitudes have improved. No matter what you have heard in the past, you should examine your options *now*.

THE CHOICE IS YOURS

It is up to you whether you want to take hormone replacement therapy after menopause. You may not need it or want it. But for those who do, it should be reassuring to know that HRT is now a safe and effective option. It won't turn the clock back, but it can work wonders when you desperately need its services. Taken correctly, it will not cause cancer and, in fact, it can help protect you against it.

You can take it for a few years and then quit when you don't need it to relieve symptoms anymore. You can take it for many years. Or you can take it for the rest of your life. However you do it, you will remain absolutely safe if you follow the rules.

The choice is up to you.

INDEX